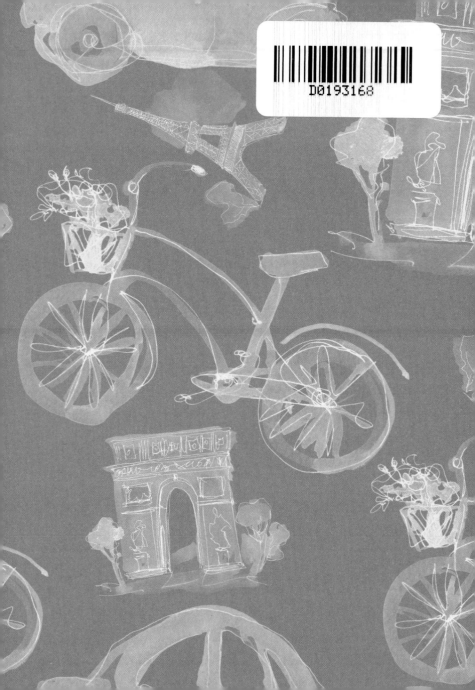

D0193168

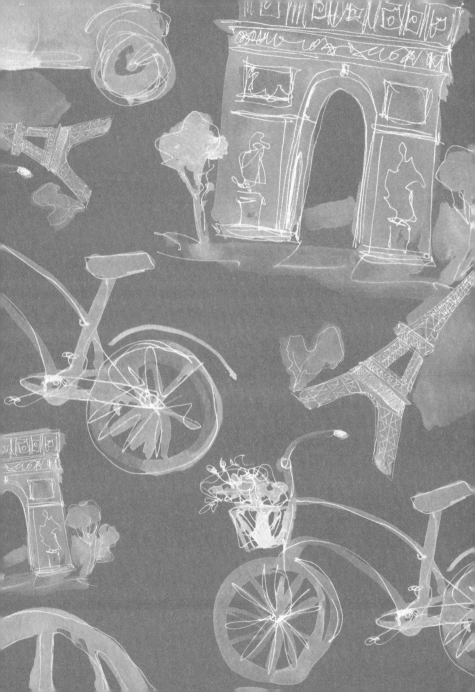

the
PARIS
Bath & Beauty Book

EMBRACE YOUR NATURAL BEAUTY
WITH TIMELESS SECRETS AND RECIPES
FROM THE FRENCH

CHRISSY CALLAHAN

RECIPES BY ANUBHA CHARAN

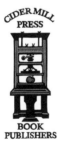

CIDER MILL PRESS

BOOK PUBLISHERS

Kennebunkport, Maine

CONTENTS

Makeup & Skincare:

The *Au Naturel* Parisian Beauty

RECIPES:

SIDEBARS:

Spa La La:

Relaxation, the Parisian Way

RECIPES:

SIDEBARS:

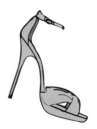

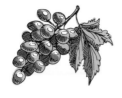

Parisian Style:
The Art of Looking Effortlessly Chic

RECIPES:

SIDEBARS:

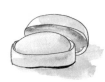
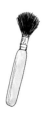

La Vie en Paris:
Lifestyle and Self-Care Secrets

RECIPES:

SIDEBARS:

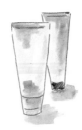

FOREWORD

Beauty is not an easy concept to define. So, what about French beauty? Even though I was born and raised in Paris, I don't know where to begin. *Oh là là...* is it even possible?

As I sat down to write this foreword, I suddenly remembered a time when an American beauty editor explained her morning beauty routine to me, which was "very simple and fast." I stopped listening when she launched into her sixth routine step, starting to feel guilty considering that I never wake up before 9 a.m., and that I only take a shower, apply a bit of hydrating cream, brush my teeth, and have an espresso (okay, three) with a cigarette (okay, three). My hair? I brush it. When I don't forget. My makeup? A good night of sleep. *Voilà.* My own morning ritual officially seemed lame.

I have read many articles about our legendary *beauté à la française*, our amazingly efficient sense of style and our typical *art de vivre*. If you could have a look at my closet, you'd think I'm the laziest girl in town. Navy or black pants and jeans; white or black tees and shirts; *marinières*; black dresses; black, navy and grey cashmeres; black heels and loafers; black and navy, bags. All from the same families: A.P.C., & Other Stories, Acne, Charvet, and a few pieces from Céline, Saint Laurent, and Chanel. I observe strict rules: dresses go with flats, and pants with heels; wear a Maison Michel hat if you need to upgrade your allure. Boring, right? Don't be fooled. The ugly truth is that I work my ass off to look this effortless. In fact, it requires mastering a lot of tricks to give off this nonchalant vibe.

Another paradox seems to be: How to eat *croissants au beurre*, and baguettes, and *fondant au chocolat* without getting fat? How to avoid the gym and stay fit? How to drink Bordeaux and smoke cigarettes without ruining your skin and your health? Well, I'll tell you: I work out five times a week, and I only indulge in croissants and bread for special occasions. I cut down on sugar to stay with my red wine, and I've learned what cosmetics are powerful enough to keep my skin glowing. And I swear to quit smoking each month.

If I had to summarize my beauty philosophy, it would be: be thoughtful, keep it simple...but be deliberate! Aim for balance to get the best of both worlds: a good cleansing routine and a good hydrating cream means you won't need foundation. Why bother using tons of products when a few will allow you to skip the superfluous? Time is precious. Time is the only real luxury in life. Time is made for re-energizing the soul and body by dancing all night long at Orphée and Le Silencio, wasting hours with friends at the bistro, reading books, listening to music, dreaming, going to your massage therapist.

In truth, our so-called "effortless charisma" is nothing more than intentional calculations based on one holy principle: enhance your natural beauty. I can't speak for all French women, but I think that more than trying to be like someone else, we deeply want to improve and reveal who we truly are. This means: chase the right red lipstick shade right across the world and you won't have to wear foundation, eye shadow, and mascara. Pledge allegiance to the best massage therapist and your body will stay firm and toned. Unearth the rare colorist who'll know how to get a chestnut hair shiny and lively. Find out the rare perfume that will adorn you like the most sophisticated dress.

That said, I have a huge confession to make. I'm totally obsessed with what I picture to be "American beauty." I was even interviewed about my great admiration for your unique flawless allure in an amazing New York-based magazine. You know what they say: "the grass is always greener on the other side of the Atlantic." I look at those impeccable American women and I think, "What is their secret to always looking so perfect? How do they manage time to wake up at dawn, go for a hardcore yoga or spin class, grab a green juice, and be at work at 8 a.m.? And with a blow-dry? *S'il vous plaît!*" Twice a year, I throw all my French classical cosmetics away (*adieu* La Roche-Posay, Esthederm, and Guerlain) and replace them with some cool and edgy American labels. It makes me feel for one second that I could be this dazzling American woman, living in Brooklyn instead of... well... me. A basic Parisian girl, smoking too much and never up before 9 a.m., in my small apartment on Montmartre. Usually, it lasts for like two weeks. Then, I remember that we are just humans after all. And that's okay. Because there may be one more secret to beauty that transcends all borders: learn to love your flaws and make them your best allies. Let them empower you. That's why we love to have static electricity in our disheveled hair (it gives you a very sexy vibe), why we're tracking spots and zits but don't fight our dark circles (they look and feel mysterious and romantic)... As devil is in the details, beauty is in personality. And storytelling.

—Julie Levoyer, Beauty Director
of *Stylist Magazine France*

"THERE MAY BE
ONE MORE SECRET
TO BEAUTY THAT
TRANSCENDS ALL
BORDERS: LEARN TO
LOVE YOUR FLAWS
AND MAKE THEM YOUR
BEST ALLIES. LET THEM
EMPOWER YOU."

MAKEUP

&

SKINCARE:

The *Au Naturel* Parisian Beauty

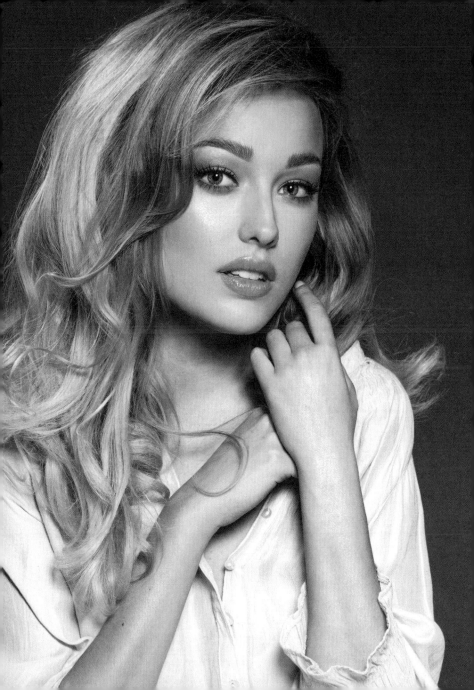

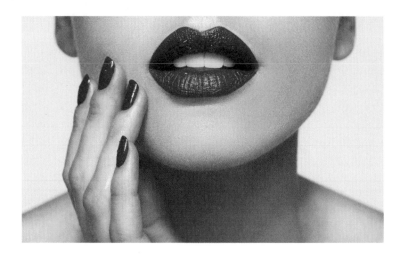

From their red lips to their flawless skin, it can seem like French women have the blueprint for makeup and skincare totally figured out. It's enough to make us mere mortals feel more than *un peu* inferior. Sure, we may have a teeny tiny complex about this. But most of the time, we just live in awe of their ability to effortlessly solve some of life's greatest beauty dilemmas.

The secret to naturally gorgeous skin? Yep, they've pretty much patented it. The recipe for a balanced, yet totally chic makeup look? It's like second nature to these gifted beauties. And yet, they do it all so seamlessly you'd swear they were all professionals.

Jealous yet? Get used to it, *ma chérie*, because Parisian women have mastered the art of looking *très belle* without overdoing their eye shadow, foundation, or lip liner—*and* they pull it off while looking naturally stunning.

Raccoon eyes and creasing eye shadow? Parisian *femmes* really don't have to worry about that; they approach all things makeup-related with a light hand. For them, the name of the makeup game is natural beauty, and the motto is "less is more."

SO, ARE FRENCH WOMEN
FREAKS OF NATURE OR ARE
THEY JUST REALLY SKILLED
AT THE ART OF BEAUTY?
WELL, IT SEEMS LIKE THEY
HAVE THEIR ROUTINES
DOWN TO A SCIENCE, AND
WE'RE ABOUT TO LET YOU
IN ON A FEW OF THEIR
ENVIABLE SECRETS.

STOCK YOUR BEAUTY BAG
LIKE A PARISIAN PRO

The contents of their makeup bags might be a bit less extensive than our laundry list of cosmetic goodies, but that just means French women know how to do more with less. And thanks to these simple yet effective beauty staples, you'll be making a Parisian beauty statement in no time.

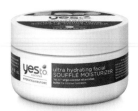

MOISTURIZER

Yes To Coconut Ultra Hydrating Facial Soufflé Moisturizer

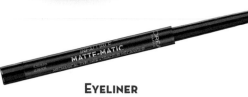

EYELINER

L'Oréal Paris Infallible® Matte-Matic Liner in Ultra Black

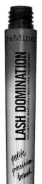
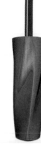

MASCARA

Lash Domination® Volumizing Mascara Petite Precision™ Brush

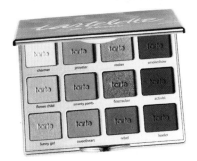

Eye Shadow

tarte tartelette 2
in bloom

Brow Gel

Urban Decay
Brow Tamer
Flexible Hold
Brow Gel

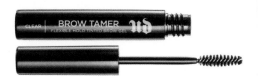

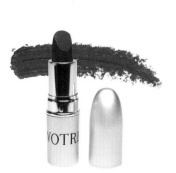

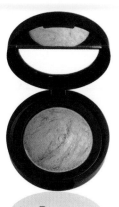

Lipstick

Votre Vu French
Kiss Moisture Riche
Lipstick in Claudia

Blush

Laura Geller Baked
Blush-n-Brighten
in Roseberry

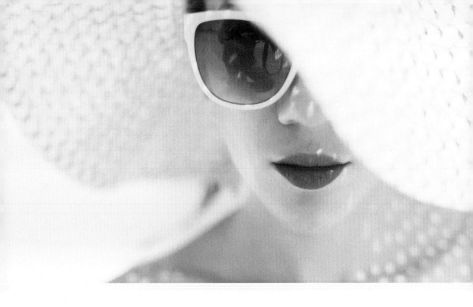

French Makeup *Philosophie*

If you've been *oohing* and *aahing* over the natural beauty look that's been reigning supreme on the runways the past few years, you'll be pleased to hear that it's a never-ending trend for Parisian women. These sage gals value toned-down makeup and subtle skin over bold colors and passing fads, and they don't like to hide their faces with cakey layers of foundation and oodles of eye shadow.

"French beauty emulates an extremely minimal look with a focus feature. French women often wear little to no face makeup paired with a saturated lip. Skin is often left extremely moisturized and bare," says Sir John, L'Oréal Paris celebrity makeup artist. "I like to describe this look as raw and undone, with a level of polish in one area—massive mascara, bold lip, etc."

Focusing on one statement feature at a time? Sounds like that saves you *beaucoup* time and lets you feel more beautiful in your own skin. In fact, Parisian women pride themselves on the ability to rock a bare face and own the features that make them distinctively beautiful. "The French makeup must be subtle and look natural with a little touch that makes you beautiful," says Muriel Vancauwen, celebrity hair and makeup artist from Paris.

And one more thing: French women don't believe makeup should "fix" their flaws. Instead, makeup is more often used as a tool to highlight their badass individual beauty. "French women are known for embracing the unique aspects of their features and do not use makeup to cover or 'correct' them," says celebrity makeup artist Roxy, who studied at one of Paris' most prestigious makeup academies.

But even if you worship the *au naturel* look, let's not kid ourselves, you're most likely not stepping out the door totally barefaced. Looking natural does take a certain degree of prep work, and French women know exactly which areas of their face to target to achieve that certain *je ne sais quoi*.

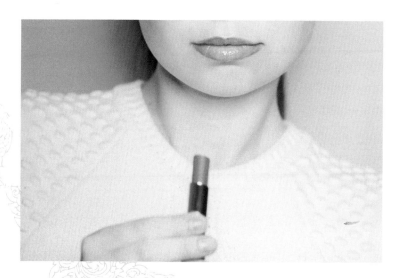

BEAUTY EXPERTS' TIPS FOR
AN AUTHENTIC PARISIAN LOOK

Coveting that classically chic Parisian makeup?
Join the club! Their barely-there beauty looks somehow
leave a *grand* impact in their wake, and leave us all
très jaloux. But thanks to these beauty experts' tips,
we no longer have to stand on the sidelines and stare.
Read on, and get ready to join the *très chic* makeup club!

1.

"Stay away from trends but instead focus on
looking like your best natural self. Own your
uniqueness and don't try to 'correct' everything
with makeup."

- CELEBRITY MAKEUP ARTIST ROXY

2.

"Do your makeup as normal, but smudge your
liner a bit, or wear your hair air dried or lived in
with a raw face and bright lip. Embrace
the perfection we love as Americans, but
make it a little grungier."

- L'ORÉAL PARIS CELEBRITY MAKEUP ARTIST SIR JOHN

3.

"In France, we are more about the look and health of the skin than the makeup coverage. It's like a painting: you need a beautiful canvas if you want the paint to look amazing."

– ANNE-CECILE CUROT, *THE FRENCH FOUNDER OF LE VISAGE SPA IN BOSTON*

4.

"Hardly use foundation and powder, which are considered unhealthy and old-looking. It means you have something to hide."

– BRIGITTE BEASSE, *CELEBRITY FACIALIST AND OWNER OF BRIGITTE BEAUTÉ IN BEVERLY HILLS*

5.

"Don't wear too much makeup or overdo your hair. Your natural beauty is what sets you apart from every other woman."

– CAMILLE PARRUITTE, *PARISIAN FOUNDER OF THE JEWELRY LINE NOUVEL HERITAGE*

Lip Balm Pour Les Lèvres

A smooth, mildly aromatic lip balm.

What Makes It Parisian?
Softens lips *pour envoyer des baisers* (for blowing kisses, of course).

What Does It Do?
This natural lip balm keeps your lips moist and protected without drying them out even more, unlike some synthetic products. Beeswax not only protects your lips, but also gives the lip balm the consistency to hold and mold to the curve of your lips, enhancing your natural beauty. Honey naturally retains water molecules, making it the perfect solution to dry and cracked lips!

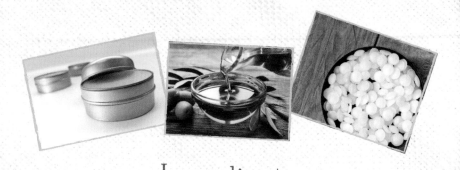

Ingredients

1 teaspoon honey
½ ounces beeswax (grated or pastilles)
4 ounces olive oil
10-15 drops of vanilla or mint extract for
flavor (optional)
1 empty lip balm tin or tube

1. In a double boiler (not a sauce pan!), melt the beeswax, then add the honey and olive oil and stir.

2. When all mixed together, add a couple drops of your favorite extract for flavor.

3. Pour your mixture into a used lip balm tin or tube (you can use a turkey baster to transport the melted mixture from the boiler to the container).

4. Let cool and solidify, then apply to freshly scrubbed lips.

Variations: You can add some drops of vitamin E, or 1 tablespoon of cocoa or shea butter, to the melting wax to enhance its pucker-packed power.

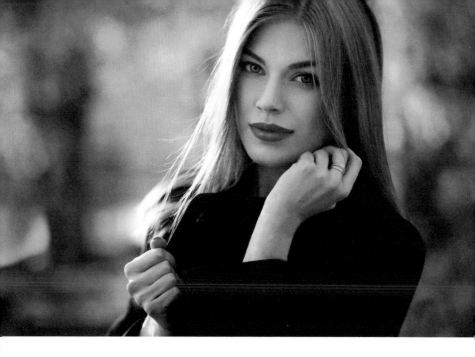

French Makeup *Essentiels*

Their *à la mode* beauty bags might not be weighed down with
a plethora of products, but Parisian women definitely have
the right tools to paint a pretty picture. And they know not to
use them all at the same time, too! Some of their must-have
makeup staples, you ask? Well, full-coverage lipstick (red, of
course!), lip balm, mascara, kohl eyeliner, brow gel, blush, and
moisturizer are mainstays in every Parisian's beauty bag.
Concealer and foundation are used sparingly, but extras like
primers, powders, bronzers, lip liners, and highlighters aren't
huge priorities for these practical *beautés*.

    With such a pared down product lineup, it should come as
no surprise that Parisian women prefer a more muted color palette.
So if you're looking to emulate their *maquillage*, go for statement

red lips, rosy lip balms, black or soft brown eyeliner, natural blushes *sans* shimmer, and minimal eye shadow—think subtle shades like violet, taupe, beige, or pastel pink. Feast your eyes on all the French makeup essentials you could need in the "Stock Your Beauty Bag Like a Parisian Pro" sidebar.

But even though they mostly color inside the lines when it comes to their makeup, that doesn't mean Parisian women aren't willing to experiment every once in a while. "Mostly classic and neutral colors are generally the way to go with French/Parisian makeup, but it's also not out of the ordinary to run into a woman wearing a striking shade of blue eyeliner or a dark plum lip acting almost as a fashion accessory to her look," Roxy says.

LESSON LEARNED: STICK TO THE BASICS THAT BRING OUT YOUR BEST FEATURES, BUT DON'T BE AFRAID OF A DARING BEAUTY STATEMENT EVERY ONCE IN A WHILE.

Whatever color or product she's wearing, you can bet that a Parisian woman likely bought it at her local *pharmacie*. The French love to shop for their makeup must-haves and beauty creams at the local pharmacy, and benefit from the high standards of product inspection in France. Natural makeup (as well as skincare) is both common and a priority for Parisians. Products are held to the highest standards of quality, and these lucky gals don't have to look far for safe beauty goodies; local *pharmacies* (as well as other boutiques) are filled with them. Some of their favorite skincare brands? Vichy, La Roche-Posay, and Caudalie. The good news for you is they're all available in the United States!

Once you've stocked your beauty bag with fun new toys, it's time to get serious about achieving the French makeup look.

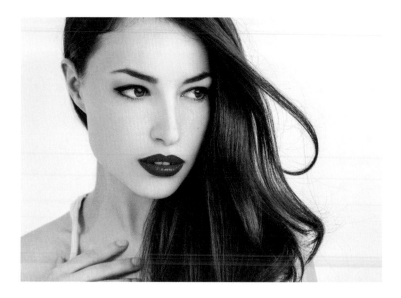

5 STEPS TO THE PERFECT PARISIAN RED LIP

Follow these five easy steps and your lips will look lusciously *rouge* la la.

1.
EXFOLIATE
using a DIY lip scrub
(see Chapter 2!)
or toothbrush

2.
APPY LIP BALM,
such as eos Visibly
Soft Lip Balm Sphere
in Vanilla Mint

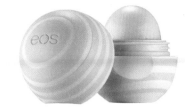

3.
APPLY LIPSTICK,
such as Burt's Bees
Lipstick in
Scarlet Soaked

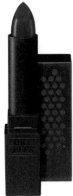

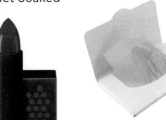

4.
BLOT LIPS
using a tissue or
blotting papers

5.
REAPPLY COLOR

Conditioning, Darkening, & Lengthening Eyelash Serum

This eyelash serum gives you lush lashes with a perfect "barely there" feeling.

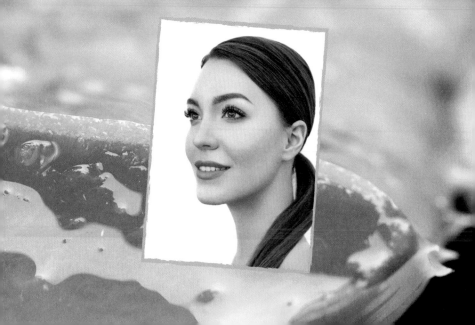

What Makes It Parisian?
Parisian women don't like loading their lashes with mascara or falsies—they'd rather stick to their own lashes, nourishing them to natural glossiness.

What Does It Do?
Castor oil thickens the lashes, while both aloe vera gel and vitamin E accelerate their length.

Ingredients
2 tablespoons castor oil
4 tablespoons vitamin E oil
2 tablespoons aloe vera gel
1 empty mascara or nail polish container
(washed well, if used)
1 mascara wand (washed well, if used)

1. Blend both the oils together.

2. Add the aloe vera gel to this mix.

3. Shake well and pour into the container.

4. Apply a light layer to lashes (or brows!) with the mascara wand every night before going to bed.

5. Follow up with a thin layer right at the lash line with a clean eyeliner brush or cotton swab; repeat daily for 6 weeks for best results.

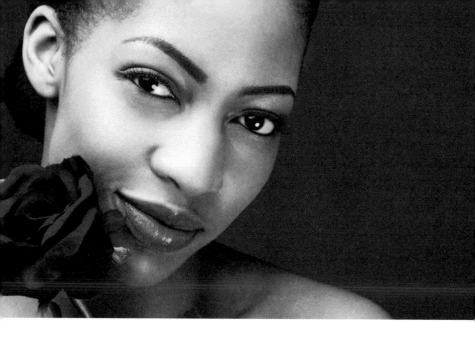

En Vogue French Makeup Tips

Why waste your time coveting Parisians' on-point makeup when you can emulate their look with a few simple tips? To start, make sure your base is clean and bright. "Perfecting the skin and understanding how to take care of your skin is a huge deal. French women have mastered this," Sir John says.

From there, *ma chérie*, remember that less is more when it comes to any product covering your skin. "If you put too much foundation on, that means you don't have a healthy life," Vancauwen says. "When women put concealer and foundation on, we mustn't see it."

Avoid a makeup meltdown by blending foundation well, avoiding heavy powders, and using product sparingly. Seriously, you never need as much as you think you do! Odds are, you'll be pretty pleased with the results: natural, hydrated skin that glows instead of hiding under a mask of products.

Speaking of using less product, Parisian women have definitely conquered the concept of "less is more" when it comes to any makeup, not just foundation. They don't feel the need to highlight their skin, contour their faces, *and* do a smokey eye. But this flair for balance doesn't stop there; it extends to their entire look.

"There is a refinement that takes place. For example, if a French woman wears a little more makeup, her hair will be pulled back," Sir John says. "If they are wearing couture or a very busy outfit, they will wear a bare face. There is a sense of balance throughout their entire look."

Want in on this balancing act? It's all about choosing which feature you want to highlight and not overdoing it. Pick *either* eyes or lips; don't use a bold color on both at the same time. This is the key to the Parisian makeup look!

IN THE END, WHATEVER FEATURE YOU CHOOSE TO HIGHLIGHT, MAKE SURE YOU DO IT WELL, BUT DON'T TAKE IT TOO SERIOUSLY. BEAUTY IS SUPPOSED TO BE FUN, AFTER ALL!

If you're lining your eyes, trace a soft line then smudge slightly to create a more lived-in effect. Or if you're going for a statement red lip, make sure you consider the shade of red you're rocking. Don't try to wear a hue just because it's *en vogue*; make sure it works for your skin tone and makes you feel confident first.

While we're at it, take trends with a grain of salt because Parisian women sure do. Naturally it's fun to watch the latest runway beauty trends every season, but none of that matters if the trending looks don't flatter the beauty staring back at you in the mirror. Focusing on looking like your best natural self and owning your look is always *à la mode* for Parisians.

THE BOTTOM LINE: PERFECTION IS PLAIN OLD BORING. BUT OWNING YOUR FLAWS AND TURNING THEM INTO SOMETHING TO BE PROUD OF? NOW THAT'S PRETTY BEAUTIFUL.

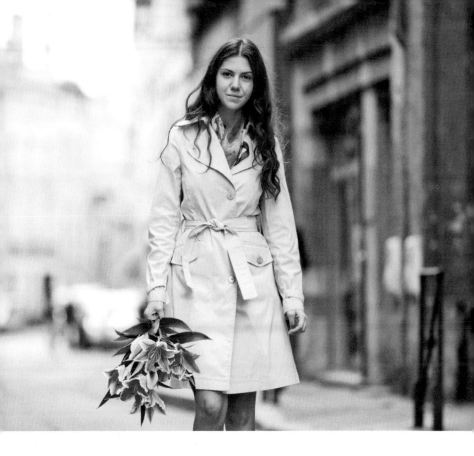

"Perfection is not the goal when a French woman approaches her makeup, but instead the desire to enhance their features with a touch of minimalism and bring them out in the most naturally beautiful way. I feel this is why so many women admire the beauty/makeup approach of French women because they generally look their best with no trace of real effort," Roxy says.

Bien sûr, Parisian women do put in effort, but they don't spend all day in front of the vanity. For them, great makeup starts with great skin.

Eye Shadow Magnifique

A lush and creamy eye shadow made with safer ingredients than your drugstore faves!

What Makes It Parisian?
The color of the eye shadow is based on how much pigment powder *you* put into the mixture, and what color *you* decide to use. Go light with pinks and browns to create that soft *naturel* French makeup look. Or enhance the brown tones to create a stunning smokey eye for evening.

What Does It Do?

Eye shadow subtly elevates your peepers. Wear it to enhance your fave mascara; brighten eyes with its soft sheen and sparkle; or go bold for the evening with a daring color choice or smokey eye. Just remember, the French look is meant to *enhance* your beauty, not cover the color and shape of your eyes.

Ingredients

4 teaspoons grated beeswax
1 teaspoon shea butter
¼ teaspoon tea tree oil
1¼ teaspoons vegetable glycerin
2 teaspoons pigment powder
in your favorite color
¼ teaspoon mica powder
1 empty eye shadow container

1. Place the beeswax and shea butter together in a glass measuring cup and melt in the microwave for about 1–1½ minutes.

2. Add the tea tree oil and glycerin to the wax mixture, using a pipette if possible.

3. Mix in the pigment powder and mica to the mixture. Stir well.

4. Transport to the eye shadow container. Let it sit for a day to set.

6 SIMPLE STEPS TO
A *TRÈS CHIC* FRENCH LOOK

It doesn't take years of training to become fluent
in the art of French beauty. With a bit of practice and
the proper tools, you can master the alluring Parisian
je ne sais quoi in a few easy steps.

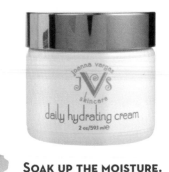

1.

SOAK UP THE MOISTURE.

Joanna Vargas Daily Hydrating Cream

COLOR INSIDE THE LINES.

BECCA Automatic Eye
Pencil in Majorca

2.

3.

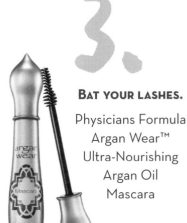

Bat your lashes.

Physicians Formula
Argan Wear™
Ultra-Nourishing
Argan Oil
Mascara

4.

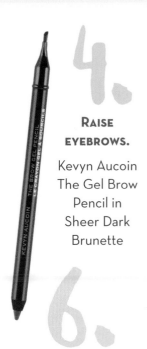

**Raise
eyebrows.**

Kevyn Aucoin
The Gel Brow
Pencil in
Sheer Dark
Brunette

6.

Get cheeky.

Paul and Joe Beauté
Powder Blush in Gamine

5.

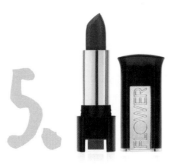

Mouth off.

FLOWER Kiss Stick High-Shine
Lip Color in Rose Bud

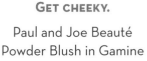

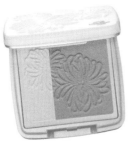

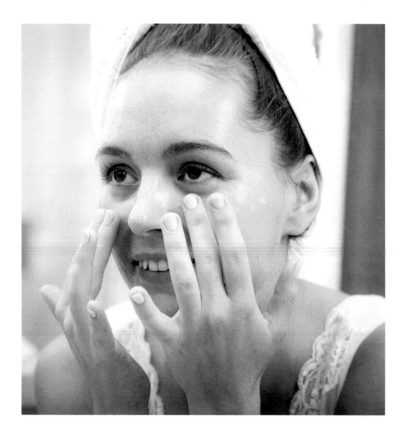

Skin and *Le Visage*

Of course, you can't paint a gorgeous picture without a clean, smooth canvas, can you? Any makeup artist worth her set of brushes knows a dedicated skincare routine is the first step to creating lust-worthy makeup looks, and Parisian women definitely got that memo. For these savvy beauties, skincare is the foundation of any beauty routine, and they spend much more time perfecting their *visage* than applying *maquillage*.

"[French women] are more into addressing a skin concern rather than hiding it with makeup," says Agnes Landau, SVP, global general manager of skincare line Darphin Paris.

After all, what's a naturally beautiful gal like you got to hide? A raw, natural look always wins out over an overdone, airbrushed one that looks nothing like your face. French ladies are much more content to let their inner beauty—flaws and all—shine while they continue on their quest for *parfait* skin.

"Taking care of the skin is extremely important as a natural radiant skin is what is considered to be beautiful in a woman," says Brigitte Beasse, celebrity facialist and owner of Brigitte BEAUTÉ in Beverly Hills.

Want skin that glows naturally like a Parisian? Press pause for a minute, and ponder these Parisian skincare secrets.

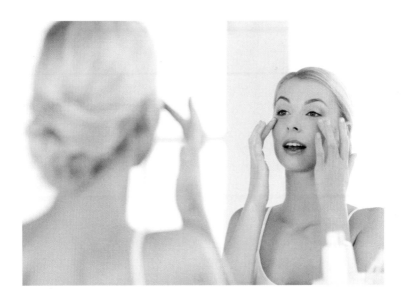

French Skincare *Essentiels*

A French woman's quest for *très belle* skin starts at an early age and involves a pretty well-oiled skincare routine. "French ladies start to take care of their skin very young. When turning 13, usually their mother takes them to a beautician who analyzes their skin and provides them with a three-step day and night skincare regimen, consisting of a cleanser, toner, and moisturizer," Beasse says.

Now that you just realized most Parisian teenagers *probably* take better care of their skin than you do on your worst days—come on, we all have those long days when we just can't bear to wash our faces, never mind slather on moisturizer—you'll be happy to hear that naturally glowing skin isn't as hard to achieve as it might seem. No seriously, it just takes a bit of commitment and a touch of *savoir-faire.*

Bien sûr, a parade of powerful products doesn't hurt either. If you took a look at their naturally beautiful *visages,* you'd think Parisian women's vanities were practically filled to the brim with skincare lotions and potions, but you'd be wrong. Sure, they love their products and inevitably inherit newbies while evolving their skincare routine over time just like any of us, but they're hardly hoarders when it comes to their priceless skincare gems. *Au contraire ma chérie,* their routine is quite simple and boils down to four to five star products.

"French women are not obsessed with skincare, but they are very particular about the products they use. That is why pharmacy brands are so popular in France: women trust their pharmacist to recommend the best products," Landau says.

So what beauty goodies top Parisians' wish list? Cleansing milks, toners, moisturizers, and eye creams win a spot in their diligent daily routine. They've also got a pretty strong love affair with micellar water, a cleanser and makeup remover that sucks up dirt, oil, and makeup without the dreaded after effect of dry skin.

But the fun doesn't stop there! Exfoliants, masks, and scrubs factor into French women's weekly rituals, and they particularly love *gommage*, a popular form of exfoliation often used on dry skin. As the years go on, women also start incorporating a serum into their routine to get a head start on the aging process.

The fight against aging is no joke for Parisian ladies, and they definitely know what they're doing when it comes to preparing for fine lines, crow's feet, and wrinkles. They start their routine early, making monthly facials the priority *du jour* in their mid-twenties, then slowly start incorporating an eye cream, serum, and mask into their routines around the same time. When their mid-thirties and early forties roll around, Parisians step up their aging game a bit with targeted facial treatments.

And even though they love a good sunny day (a subtle tan adds a natural glow and lets you skip foundation, after all!), French women are always vigilant about applying sunscreen, especially while on vacation.

What about the ingredients in all these skincare gems, you ask? Well, French women look for quality ingredients—they love natural ones—and look for a pleasant consistency too. "The texture has to feel good: the sensation of well-being—*bien être*—acts as a huge factor in French cosmetics selling points. French women trust and respect major French brands because making cosmetics is strongly embedded in our traditions and culture," Beasse says.

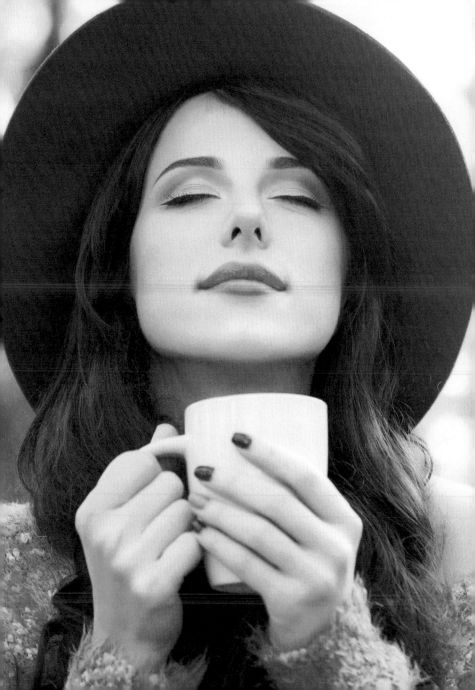

TIP:
Don't wear too much
makeup or overdo your hair.
Your natural beauty is what
sets you apart from every
other woman.

ANTI-PUFFINESS UNDER-EYE MASK

This under-eye mask feels super refreshing... the perfect antidote to tired eyes!

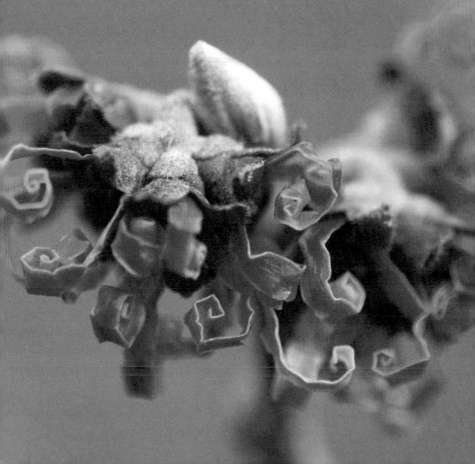

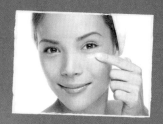

What Makes It Parisian?
It's gentle and natural. And it does away with the need for under-eye concealer or illuminator.

What Does It Do?
Witch hazel has a refreshing, astringent effect on the skin, helping deflate under-eye circles. Similarly, celery is packed with over a dozen anti-inflammatory agents, including apigenin, which is an integral part of several anti-inflammatory drugs.

Ingredients
2 celery stalks (or 2 tablespoons celery juice)
1 green tea bag
2 cups witch hazel
1 tablespoon glycerin

1. Puree the celery stalks and strain the juice.

2. Place the teabag in a glass beaker.

3. Heat witch hazel until hot and pour it on top of the teabag.

4. Let the tea infuse for 2-3 minutes, then remove the teabag.

5. Add celery juice and glycerin.

6. Saturate a gauze pad and place over the eyes for 15 minutes.

7. Keep refrigerated; discard if the mixture becomes cloudy.

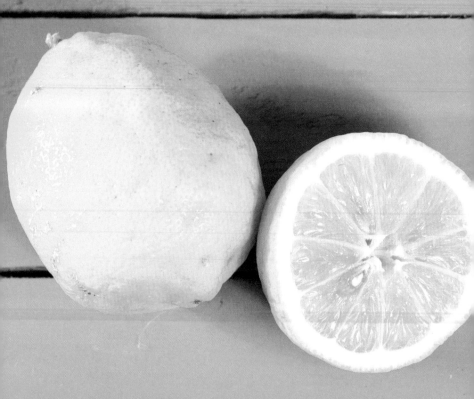

Lemon Facial Scrub

The glow of gold adds a touch of luxury to this most basic and essential of beauty rituals.

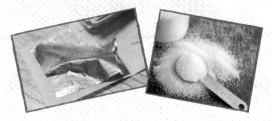

What Makes It Parisian?

This is based on a traditional French beauty recipe dating from the late 1700s.

What Does It Do?

Lemon juice is loaded with citric acid, which helps bleach away dark spots, age spots, and other kinds of hyperpigmentation. It also absorbs excessive oiliness and deep cleans the pores without drying out the skin. Sugar makes for an effective natural scrub, and the gold leaf peps up the skin's natural resources to guard against premature aging.

Ingredients

½ lemon
1 teaspoon granulated sugar
¼ sheet gold leaf

1. Using a sharp knife, scoop a hole in the lemon and fill it with granulated sugar. The hole should run through approximately half the lemon.

2. Cover the hole with a light seal of the gold leaf.

3. Very lightly roast the lemon over a stove or grill.

4. Squeeze the juice from the lemon and apply it to your face; leave on for half an hour, then rinse well.

Get Skin Like A *Parisienne*

So you want skin as supple as a Parisian, huh? Well *ma chérie*, it all boils down to a few key tips. To start, let's look at the obvious, shall we? One of the simplest steps in your routine—cleansing—is also one of the most neglected, and a lot of us have it all wrong.

It's a nasty cycle, really—wear *beaucoup* makeup, don't wash said makeup off before bed, break out, cover up breakouts with more makeup, repeat. If you think you can get away with going to bed with your makeup on, or just want to splash a touch of water on your face, think again.

"Water doesn't wash; water rinses. You need something to wash, an emulsion, it doesn't need to be very foaming," says Anne-Cecile Curot, the French founder of Le Visage Spa in Boston.

Washing their makeup off is high priority for French women, because they know how intimately related skincare and makeup are, so do what you have to do to summon the energy to wipe it off at night. Invest in some makeup wipes or find a cleanser you'll *want* to use. Either way, just wash!

If you're really committed and have five extra seconds, spray on a toner after cleansing (morning or night). Parisian women swear by toners and it's easy to find one that works for your skin type and won't strip your skin.

Parisian gals even take things one step further by using their favorite washcloths to get a closer cleanse—gentle glove washcloths are very popular in the country!

It's these simple touches that make their skincare routine all the more luxurious and relaxing, even though it's otherwise low-maintenance.

"French women, we do less. We do maybe a mask once a week. But we take the time for simple steps," Curot says.

IT'S THESE SIMPLE TOUCHES THAT MAKE THEIR SKINCARE ROUTINE ALL THE MORE LUXURIOUS AND RELAXING, EVEN THOUGH IT'S OTHERWISE LOW-MAINTENANCE.

And the fact that they stop to enjoy the process is pretty enviable in and of itself! So next time you do a face mask, stop and grab your favorite magazine for a few minutes instead of running around the house checking items off your to-do list. Sometimes, it just feels darn good to forget about multitasking for a second, and Parisian women definitely prefer to savor their skincare routines rather than rush the process.

It's that leisurely, relaxed attitude towards beauty that gives Parisian gals the patience to look for long-term beauty benefits instead of quick fixes. Translation? Swap some of your instant beauty gratification for some long-term patience if you're aiming for a uniquely French look.

Finally, keep it simple, lady! Just like with makeup, less is more when it comes to skincare, and all you really need is a small stash of products to get your skin on the road to glow town.

ROCK FLAWLESS PARISIAN SKIN WITH THESE 6 SKINCARE SAVIORS

In the game of skincare, Parisians always play to win. Gorgeous skin is the foundation of their beauty philosophy, and their routines are jam packed with skin-nourishing steps that cater to *le visage*. Want to model your own routine off these skincare sages? Try working these gems into your routine.

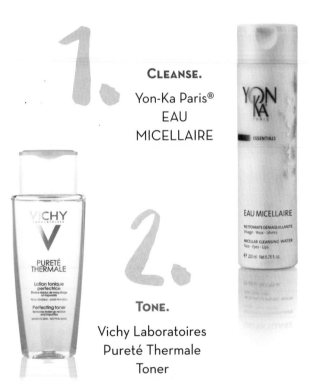

CLEANSE.

Yon-Ka Paris®
EAU
MICELLAIRE

TONE.

Vichy Laboratoires
Pureté Thermale
Toner

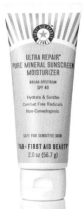

3.

Moisturize.

First Aid Beauty® Ultra Repair® Pure Mineral Sunscreen Moisturizer SPF 40

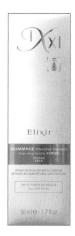

4.

Exfoliate.

IXXI Elixir One-Step Gentle Scrub

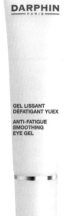

5.

Refresh.

Darphin Anti-Fatigue Smoothing Eye Gel

6.

Treat.

SkinCeuticals C E Ferulic®

ANTI-ACNE SERUM

This acne fighter can be slightly stinky, so you may want to go at it when you're alone!

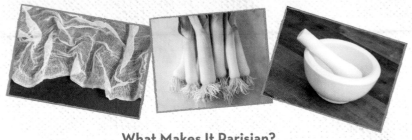

What Makes It Parisian?

Parisian women are fanatics about classic beauty recipes –
like this one, which dates from the 1700s – that have
stood the test of time and have been passed down
by word of mouth through the generations.

What Does It Do?

Leeks contain potent doses of quercetin, an antioxidant
that is a recognized acne-buster and scar lightener.

Ingredients

1 houseleek floret
1 teaspoon rubbing alcohol
Strainer or cheesecloth
Mortar and pestle

1. Pound the houseleek in the mortar, then squeeze out
its juice.

2. Strain away the leek and keep the juice.

3. Pour a few drops of rubbing alcohol on the juice;
it will turn milky.

4. Apply this liquid on acne spots and scarred areas nightly.

Traditional French Face Butter

This truly luxe recipe will give you buttery soft skin like you wouldn't believe!

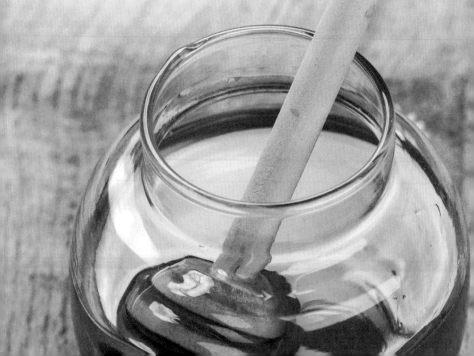

What Makes It Parisian?

It's a historic French recipe that dates all the way back to the 1600s.

What Does It Do?

The oils and beeswax melt into skin to nourish it from within. Onion juice is packed with antioxidants, B-complex, sulfur, and vitamins A, C, and E, so it's antiseptic, anti-bacterial, anti-microbial, and anti-inflammatory. It also steps up circulation, boosts dull skin, and protects against UV rays and environmental toxins.

Ingredients

4 ounces almond oil
3 ounces extra virgin olive oil
1 ounce beeswax
2 tablespoons onion juice
10 drops vanilla essential oil

1. Place the almond oil, olive oil, and wax in a heavy bottomed pan and warm just enough to melt the wax.

2. Add the onion juice and vanilla essential oil.

3. Keep stirring the mixture to keep the ingredients from separating; be especially careful about the onion juice because it will start lumping if the mixture gets too hot.

4. Cool this creamy concoction and massage it into your face, neck, arms, and feet at bedtime.

5. Leave on overnight, then use a gentle face wash, toner, or moisturizer in the morning.

Marie Antoinette's Face Mask

*This deep cleansing face mask
is the perfect way to detox
your skin.*

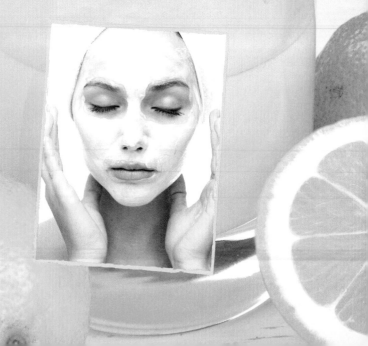

What Makes It Parisian?

This is our take on Marie Antoinette's personal favorite from more than two centuries ago.

What Does It Do?

Cognac stimulates circulation, tightens pores, and brightens the complexion; eggs repair skin tissue, help optimize the moisture within skin cells, slow down premature aging, and bust acne-causing bacteria; lemons are natural exfoliants that remove the top layer of dead skin cells, while simultaneously lightening age spots and hyper-pigmentation; and milk is a potent deep cleanser.

Ingredients

2 teaspoons cognac (or vodka, in a pinch)
$\frac{1}{3}$ cup dry milk powder
1 egg white
Juice of 1 lemon

1. Pour all ingredients into a blender and process into a smooth paste. (If you don't have a blender, mix well by stirring with a fork or wire whisk in a glass bowl.)

2. Put a large dollop of this paste aside and apply the rest on your face; allow it to dry (approximately 15 minutes).

3. Use the remaining paste to remove the mask by rubbing in small circles with fingertips.

4. Finally, rinse your face thoroughly with warm water and pat dry. End with your favorite moisturizer.

5 WAYS TO AGE GRACEFULLY
COMME LES FRANÇAIS

To say Parisian women think early and often about the aging process is an understatement. These skin *savants* start fighting against fine lines and wrinkles at a young age, and have amassed a host of tricks worth copying. Want to learn from their wise ways? Follow these tips!

1.

FIND TIME FOR FACIALS.

Glowing skin can take a village, and finding an aesthetician you trust to guide your skin on the path to agelessness is a top Parisian priority.

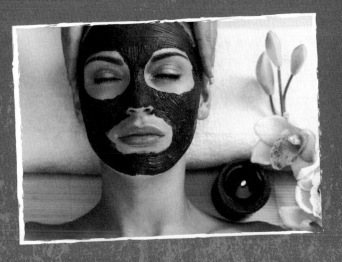

2.

EMBRACE YOUR NATURAL BEAUTY.

French women strive to look natural and celebrate their unique beauty, so it's not surprising that they find it easy to embrace their changing face as the years go on.

3.

START A ROUTINE EARLY.

The French start their anti-aging routine early so they can get ahead of the aging process before it catches up to them. Doing so also saves you from relying on drastic measures later on.

4.

COMMIT TO YOUR GOALS.

Parisians don't have an extensive skincare routine, but they do commit to the one they have, and all that dedication and consistency definitely pays off over time.

5.

BUT DON'T RUSH THE PROCESS.

There's a time and a place for everything and every step of the anti-aging process has its proper spot in the timeline of life. Make sure you're using the right products for your age, and your skin will thank you for it!

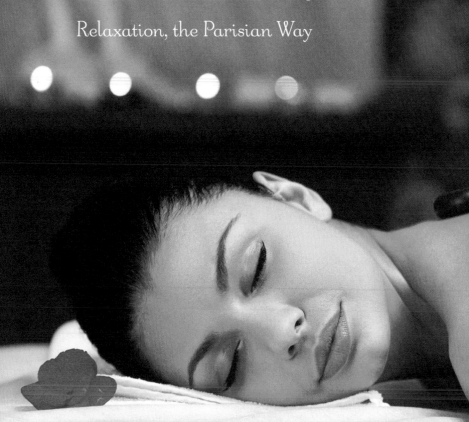

SPA
LA LA:

Relaxation, the Parisian Way

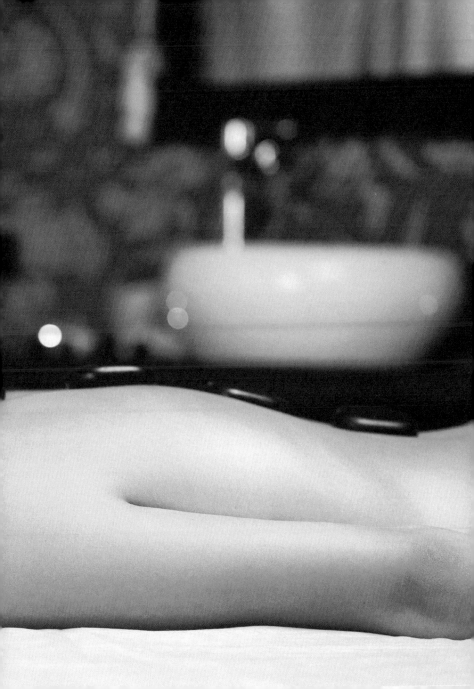

Paris is known for its *magnifique* culture, its *délicieux* food, and its *fantastique* fashion, but Parisians are also pretty famous for their lust-worthy approach to relaxation. And when these ladies kick back, they sure do know how to do it right.

FROM REGULAR SPA VISITS FOR BODY-BEAUTIFYING TREATMENTS AND SKIN-PERFECTING FACIALS TO LOW-KEY HAIR AND NAIL MAINTENANCE ROUTINES, PARISIAN WOMEN HAVE CORNERED THE MARKET ON PROPER SPA PAMPERING.

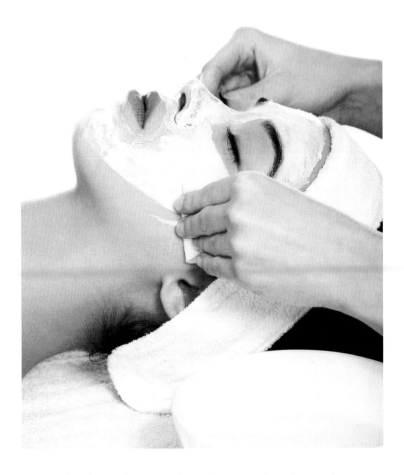

But their leisurely approach to downtime doesn't stop there; *les Parisiennes* have a wealth of ideas for other relaxing ways to spend their free time. Whether they're taking it easy with a glass of wine or saying Namaste at a yoga class, Parisian women are experts at the art of leisure.

SPA *CHEZ VOUS*: HOW TO CREATE
AN AT-HOME FRENCH SPA EXPERIENCE

Who says you need to visit an actual spa to reap all
the relaxing benefits of one? With a bit of creativity and a few
luxurious products, you can create a genuine French spa
experience in the comfort of your own home for a fraction
of the price! These winning formulas will get you started.

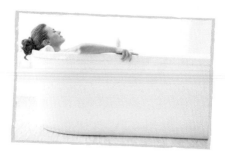

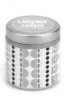 ### SET THE *SCÈNE*

One of the best parts of the spa experience?
The delicious smells! Set the scene for a luxurious
experience with a mix of scents sure to please the senses.

Paddywax®
Kaleidoscope
Collection
Lavender and
Cassis Candle

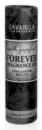

Lavanila
Forever
Fragrance
Oil in Vanilla
Grapefruit

2. ABOUT FACE

There's no need for pricey facials when you've got all the DIY skin aids you could want in your personal beauty cabinet.

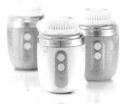 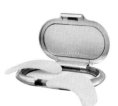 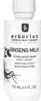

Clarisonic®
Mia Fit

Talika Eye
Therapy Patch

Erborian
Ginseng Milk

3. BODY *BEAUTÉ*

From serious slimming scrubs to magnificent massages, *les Parisiennes* sure know how to keep their bodies beautiful at the spa.

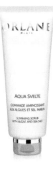 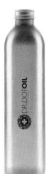 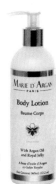

Orlane
Aqua
Svelte
Slimming
Scrub

Dr. Dot
Massage Oil
Lavender
Scent

Marie
D'Argan Paris
Body Lotion

4. Nailing It

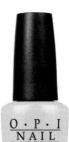

Large and in charge polishes
aren't exactly their favorites,
but neutrals, reds, and light hues
sure do color Parisians pretty.

OPI Nail Lacquer in "Stop I'm Blushing!"

5. Magnifique Manes

Parisian beauties are *très* low-key when it comes to
their hair routine, but they always treat their tresses
to luxurious masks.

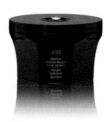

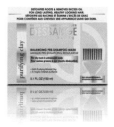

Oribe Signature
Moisture
Masque

Dessange Paris
Purifying Clay Balancing
Pre-Shampoo Mask

Bons Spas de Jour: Parisian Day Spas

Even talented DIY divas know their own limits, and French *femmes* know when it's time to seek out the expertise of beauty pros. The European beauties adore frequent spa visits to supplement their at-home beauty routines, and most opt for frequent deep cleansing facials and monthly waxing.

Since they're regulars, *les Parisiennes* love to pick a great day spa for their frequent services, then they head to more targeted spas to enjoy specialty and trendy treatments. "Right now the rage in Paris is for Chinese massage that really helps you with stress and relaxes you," says Marie-Laure Fournier, a Parisian publicist based in New York City.

Day spa trips are mostly accomplished *toute seule*, but Parisian ladies love to venture out to specialty or destination spas with friends or significant others.

LIP SCRUB

A lip scrub that smells and tastes
heavenly? You might not want
to wash it off!

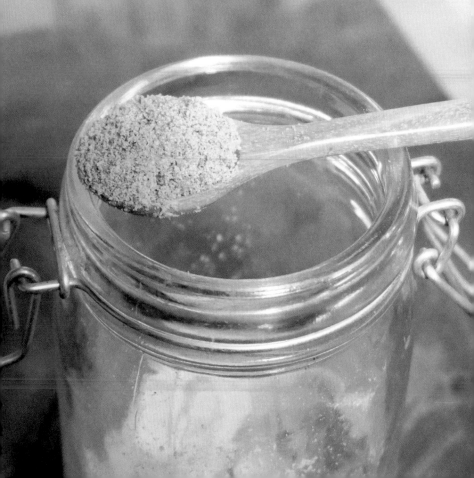

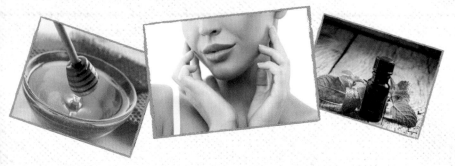

What Makes It Parisian?
Because you can't put on that signature red lipstick with less-than-perfect lips, right?

What Does It Do?
This scrub will slough all the dry, dead, and patchy skin off your lips to keep them soft, smooth, and pretty.

Ingredients
1 tablespoon fine brown sugar
1 tablespoon jojoba oil or olive oil
1 tablespoon honey
3 drops peppermint essential oil (optional)

1. Combine the ingredients in a small glass jar and give them a really good stir.

2. To use, lightly massage into the lips with circular motions, then rinse off.

3. Finish off by using your favorite lip moisturizer.

Spécialité Spa Treatments

Is there anything more relaxing than a day of pampering at the spa? *Non!* But for French women, the spa offers much more than a relaxing haven; it's also a destination for getting serious about their beauty routines. Parisians spa it up for all sorts of reasons—relaxation (massages), beautification (facials), or health reasons (slimming treatments). And many of the treatments they seek out are quite unique!

Take lymphatic drainage, for instance. This detoxifying, energizing massage technique uses gentle motions to drain your lymphatic system of toxins and other junk you don't necessarily want to keep — like water you might be retaining.

"In France, we'll have people once or twice a week come to the spa and get lymphatic drainage. It's very gentle; it's all about draining the lymphatic system," says Anne-Cecile Curot, the French founder of Le Visage Spa in Boston. "Whereas here nobody asks for it."

Another Parisian spa specialty you don't see too often in America? Bust treatments. Whether they just had a baby, recently finished breastfeeding, are about to have plastic surgery (breast reduction or augmentation), or just want to beautify their busts, women head to the spa for bust treatments to make their skin *un peu* more elastic. "The goal of this treatment is to really tone, firm, and lift the skin," Curot reveals.

Sagging, uneven skin tone, lines, and sun damage are all targeted with these facial-like treatments. Cleansing, toning, exfoliation, masks, serums, and even extractions are all a part of the process, and clients keep up the effects of their treatments by applying bust creams at home.

Les française also occasionally venture out for a weekend of thalassotherapy—therapeutic spa treatments involving seawater, seaweed, algae, etc.—and a hammam—Turkish bath—from time to time.

LESSON LEARNED: DON'T SHY AWAY FROM OUT-OF-THE-BOX SPA TREATMENTS. SOMETIMES, THE WACKIER THEY SOUND, THE MORE BENEFICIAL THEY ACTUALLY ARE!

And every once in a while, don't forget to treat yourself to splurge treatments you might not otherwise try (like a bust treatment). You don't ever need an excuse to indulge; you deserve it, girl!

Stretch Mark Serum

This body paste may seem a little sticky and runny but that's a small price to pay for flawless skin post-baby, or after any significant weight change.

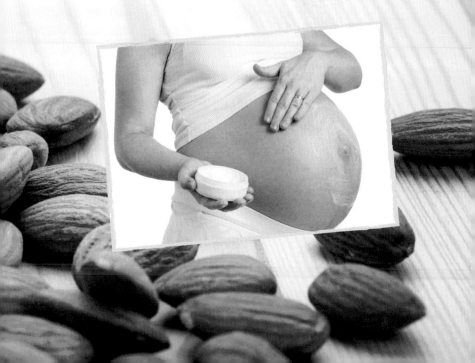

What Makes It Parisian?
Parisian women take their skincare, cellulite, and stretch marks very, very seriously!

What Does It Do?
Lemon's natural acids gently remove dead skin cells and lighten scars without stripping the skin of its natural oils. The calcium and minerals in almond oil, smooth and soften skin without leaving a greasy residue. Honey helps lighten scars and deflate bumps by boosting skin's healing and regenerating capabilities. Plus, it prevents the stringy kind of collagen that creates scar tissue. Honey also and restores hydration and elasticity to the deepest layers of your skin.

Ingredients
2 tablespoons lemon juice
2 tablespoons sweet almond oil
2 tablespoons honey

1. Pour the sweet almond oil and honey into a glass bowl; mix well.

2. Add the lemon juice; mix again until all the ingredients are well-blended.

3. Rub this mixture into stretch marks.

4. Leave on for 5-10 minutes, then rinse away.

5. Repeat daily.

PARIS SPAS TOTALLY WORTH BLOWING YOUR TRAVEL BUDGET

A trip to Paris is an indulgence in and of itself, but there should always be room in the travel budget for a little bit of pampering. After all, the city is filled with luxe spas worth blowing your travel budget, like these tempting locations.

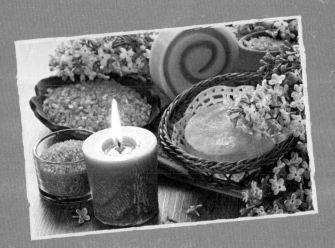

Spa Le Bristol By La Prairie

Looking for the head-to-toe spa works and a scenic backdrop to boot? Check yourself into Spa Le Bristol By La Prairie. Located on the Rue du Faubourg Saint-Honoré, this relaxing haven offers face, body, and hair services, and you can even dip your toes (or your whole body) into the hammam experience in the spa's famed Russian Room.

FOUR SEASONS HOTEL GEORGE V SPA

Conveniently located right near the Champs-Élysées, this luxurious spa is perfect for the sleepy shopper or tired traveler who just needs a little TLC. Signature treatments with a unique Parisian flair and a simply stunning atmosphere make this spa a must-try for Francophiles everywhere.

INSTITUT ORLANE PARIS

Looks like the brand doesn't just create great beauty products! Orlane also has an Institute, located in the 16th arrondissement. Here, and at other locations throughout the world, lucky ladies can experience Orlane's exclusive massage method; a hair salon; face, body, and nail services; an interior garden; and more.

SPA MY BLEND BY CLARINS

Also located right near the Champs-Élysées, Spa My Blend by Clarins (housed inside the snazzy Le Royal Monceau – Raffles Paris hotel) practically oozes luxury (in the most glamorous way, of course) with its crisp white decor. The chic space features a 23-meter infinity pool, a laconium room and sauna, a hammam, and a fitness room.

MANDARIN ORIENTAL PARIS SPA

Add this one to your spa bucket list, loves! The lavish Mandarin Oriental clocks in at an impressive 9,700 square feet, which means there's more than enough room for their private and couples suites, 14 meter lap pool, oriental herbal steam room, and fitness and wellness center.

Seasonal Spa Treatments

To every treatment, there is a season, so to speak. In other words, the type of treatments French women get at the spa can vary based on the time of year. "It all depends on the season. In wintertime Parisian ladies opt for facial cares that protect their skin. In spring, they will worry about their bodies, their thinness and therefore will head for detox and slimming cares," explains Orlane General Manager Raffaella.

Fighting the battle against pesky cellulite is high on the priority list of *les Parisiennes*, and since they don't particularly love working out, they adore experimenting with different sprays, creams, and gels to prevent and treat this annoying beauty reality.

Cellulite-fighting machines and traditional methods like the *palper rouler* massage are two other weapons Parisians like to keep in their beauty arsenal. "In France we are obsessed with weight, so anything that can help you losing weight is always welcomed," Fournier says.

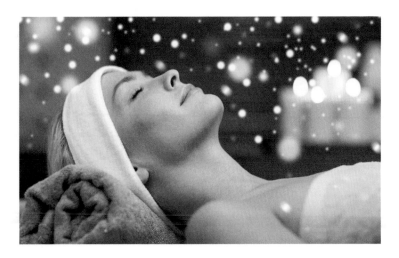

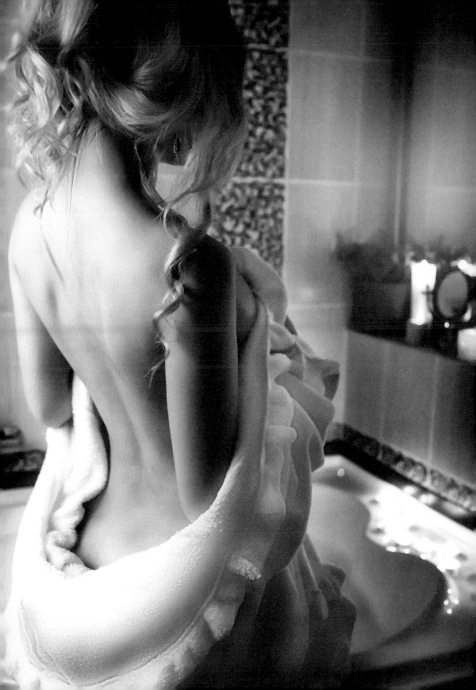

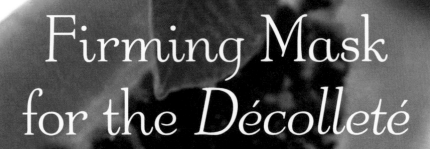

Firming Mask
for the *Décolleté*

This mask may be a little messy and drippy, but try it and get ready to watch your skin glow!

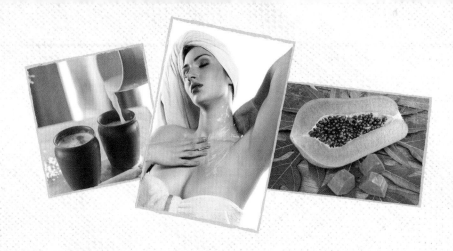

What Makes It Parisian?
Because Parisian women recognize that skincare goes beyond the face.

What Does It Do?
Papaya and buttermilk are both perfect for tightening and nourishing collagen-hungry skin.

Ingredients
4 tablespoons of fresh papaya, smashed
2 tablespoons of buttermilk

1. Blend together the papaya and buttermilk.

2. Apply this mixture on your breasts; leave for 15-20 minutes.

3. Wash off with lukewarm water.

Relaxation à *Paris*

The spa is by far our favorite place to decompress, but alas, we're not made of money, so finding other ways to unwind is always a smart idea.

From peaceful Pilates to the great outdoors and a simple glass of wine, French *femmes* have all kinds of ideas for taking it easy at the end of a long day.

FRENCH *FEMMES* HAVE ALL KINDS OF IDEAS FOR TAKING IT EASY AT THE END OF A LONG DAY.

Most ladies like to switch things up and vary their method of relaxation, depending on their mood. "To relax I think it is definitely a glass of wine at the end of the day or some free time on a beach or at the mountain," Leonor Greyl president Caroline Greyl says.

Elisabeth Holder, co-president of Ladurée US, also likes to keep her leisure options open: "Personally I do yoga and keep telling myself Rome was not built in one day! Having a sense of priorities helps me. A long sauna as well, a glass of wine, a swim. It depends where I am, but I have learned to take care of myself and relax."

Parisian women are definitely experts at carving out little bits of time to relax doing their favorite activities. "It is essential to provide breaks, whether for meditation, or for yoga; but also time for family and friends, to go to the countryside or to the beach," Raffaella explains.

"We have always been into candles, not only for aromatherapy, but for the luscious and sexy aspect of it. At the end of the day, remember a woman always looks her best with candlelight," Fournier says.

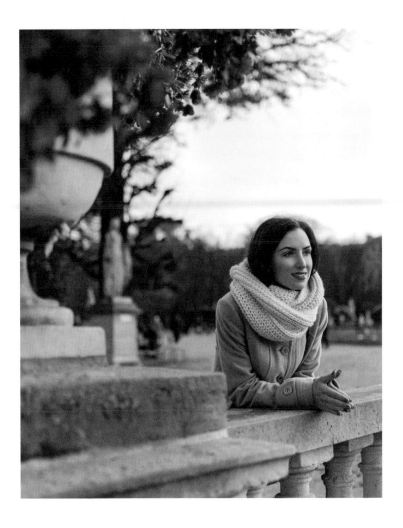

The end goal, of course, is to refuel from the hustle and bustle of daily life, but certain Parisian relaxation tools also have the added bonus of making you look and feel even more beautiful.

CERTAIN PARISIAN RELAXATION TOOLS HAVE THE ADDED BONUS OF MAKING YOU LOOK AND FEEL EVEN MORE BEAUTIFUL.

Au Naturel Mane Moves

Ok, so we've practically drooled over their serene spa trips and creative relaxation methods, but how do French women approach one of American women's favorite guilty pleasures: hair? Well, you'll be pleased to hear that Parisian gals have some pretty shareable tress tips.

Like their American *amies*, Parisian ladies want healthy manes, but they take a somewhat more *au naturel* approach when it comes to their beloved strands, especially when it comes to day-to-day styling. "French women, we don't really blow dry our hair. We like to get haircuts, we like to get maybe highlights or lowlights, but we are not obsessed with our hair," Curot says.

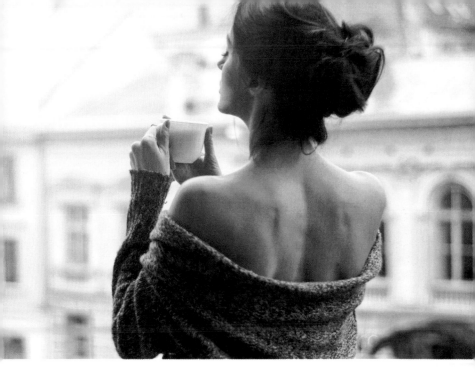

PARISIAN LADIES WANT
HEALTHY MANES, BUT THEY
TAKE A SOMEWHAT MORE
AU NATUREL APPROACH
WHEN IT COMES TO THEIR
BELOVED STRANDS.

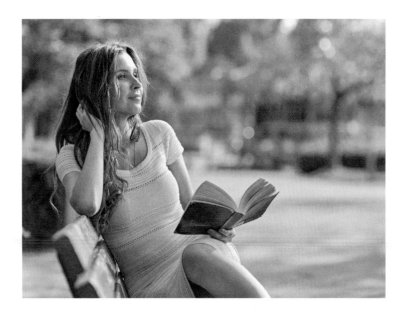

Guess what that means? If air-drying is your one true love, but you usually feel too lazy forgoing a blow-dry, go ahead and skip out on the heat styling for a naturally wavy, authentically Parisian look. They love to let their natural waves run free and as an added bonus, it can be pretty fun to upgrade toned down natural locks with a cute little accessory (try a snazzy elastic or a barrette). "We want something easy. We don't want to wake up two hours early," Curot reveals.

Another easy way to upgrade your hair *à la* stylish French women? Refreshing it with your signature scent. "This is the ultimate of how French women add extra allure and sexiness to their already naturally chic hair," says Kérastase Paris Artistic Director Nina Dimachki. "If your hair tends to get oily, spray over dry shampoo. If your hair is naturally dry, spray before applying a moisturizing balm to the hair."

Stress-Free Routine

You can forget about daily shampooing if you're going for the Parisian look; French ladies tend to wash their hair two to three times a week. Sounds pretty difficult to do when you're used to a more regimented hair routine, but your hair will love you for it in the end.

"Less shampooing is great for the hair because it allows the natural oils from your scalp to keep your hair moisturized," Cortney Peck, stylist at Boston's Jeffrey Lyle Salon, explains. "Dry shampoo is good to have on hand while adapting to not washing hair so much. Brushing hair daily also spreads oils to ends instead of leaving it sitting on roots."

Parisian ladies keep their at-home routines low-key, and they also aren't married to their salon schedules. Those with hard-to-maintain cuts make a date with their stylist every five to seven weeks, but otherwise, many women only head to the salon four times a year to refresh their look.

The same *laissez-faire* attitude goes for their hair color. "French women like their hair to look natural. If it is colored, it needs to be a color that suits their complexion and eye color," French hair colorist Christophe Robin explains.

That means saying *au revoir* to high maintenance hues and frequent trips to the salon, and *bonjour* to color sessions every six weeks or so. "When they go blonder, they won't go blonde from the roots but will layer blonde on the ends. They don't want to always have to be touching up their roots," Robin says.

Hearing the hallelujah chorus sing, yet? Parisians' relaxed attitude towards hair care is certainly something to get giddy about. So are their pared-down product routines.

Le Shampooing

Une bouteille biologique de shampooing! *A non-fussy shampoo made at home.*

What Makes It Parisian?

This easy-to-make at-home shampoo is made from all-natural ingredients, and it helps you achieve a laid-back French approach to hair styling. Add drops of lavender for a classic French scent.

What Does It Do?

At-home shampoo offers a healthy, environmentally-friendly alternative to most commercial shampoos. Generic shampoo tends to have ingredients meant to clog the pores on your head and prevent your body from naturally releasing oils.

Keep in mind: often people experience greasier hair than normal after switching to an all-natural shampoo, because their hair is releasing all the excess grease (*dégueulasse!*). This will stop in about a week's time, revealing beautiful, shiny, and *healthy* hair! Plus – happy pores.

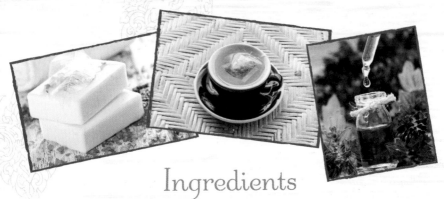

Ingredients

½ cup green tea
½ cup Castile soap
2 tablespoons coconut oil
Pure lavender essential oil

1. Boil water and pour ½ cup over a green tea bag. If your coconut oil is solidified, add 2 tablespoons into the tea mixture so that it melts into the tea. Let cool with tea bag left in.

2. Remove the tea bag. In a tight-lidded container (whatever at-home container you intend on keeping your shampoo in) pour in the tea and coconut oil mixture. Add the Castile soap.

3. Based on your own preference, add drops of the pure lavender essential oil into the shampoo. Try 5-10 drops, but don't overdo the strength of the scent!

4. Ingredients will separate, so shake before use. Best results if used with an all-natural conditioner such as coconut oil or apple cider vinegar.

TIP:
At the end of the day,
remember a woman always
looks her best with candlelight.

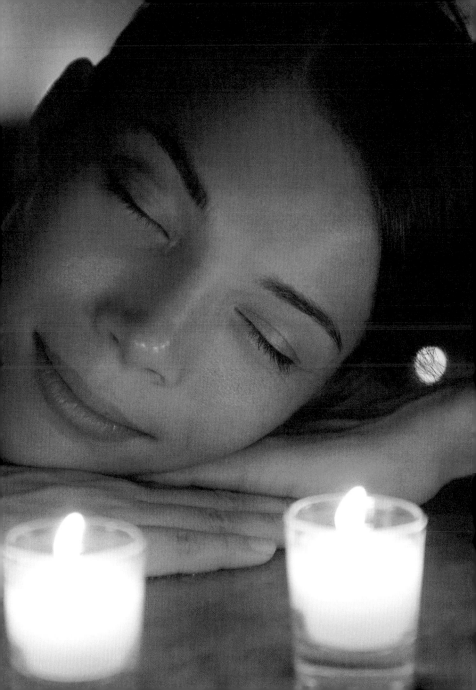

Lavender and Coconut Milk Hair Mask

Both lavender oil and coconut milk are great at replenishing hydration without weighing down your strands. Bonus: they'll make your hair smell amazing!

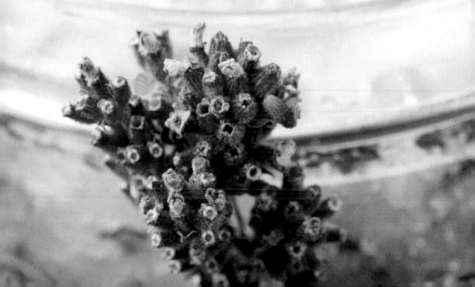

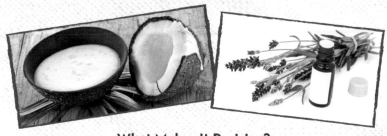

What Makes It Parisian?

Because it's *lavender*! And because French women love soft, naturally glossy hair that doesn't need to be subjected to styling tools!

What Does It Do?

The lavender oil and coconut milk are perfect for softening and adding gloss to dry and brittle strands. This recipe makes enough for shoulder-length hair; there should be just enough to coat your strands lightly without dripping. If you have longer hair you may scale up the volume accordingly, maintaining the one-to-one ingredient ratio.

Ingredients

1 teaspoon lavender oil
1 teaspoon fresh (or canned) full-fat coconut milk

1. Combine the lavender oil and coconut milk.

2. Massage the mixture into dry hair before you hit the bed; leave the mask in your hair while you sleep.

3. Simply wash and condition your hair as normal in the morning . . . you won't believe the texture!

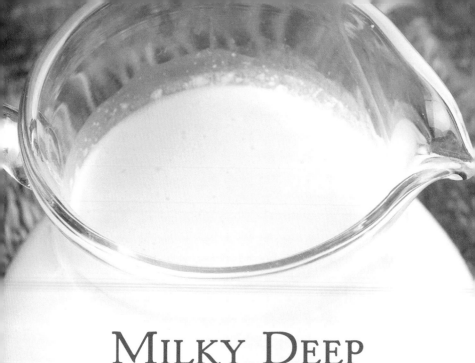

MILKY DEEP CONDITIONER FOR HAIR

Deep conditioner infused with milk adds body and shine to fine or lifeless hair, making for super-glossy locks.

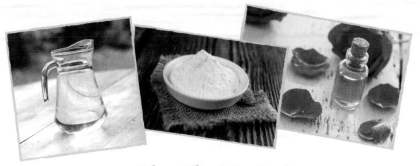

What Makes It Parisian?

It gives the effortless, cool girl hair texture that Parisian women are renowned for across the world!

What Does It Do?

Milk is loaded with minerals and vitamins that nourish and heal the hair follicle from the inside out.

Ingredients

Half a cup of dry milk powder
Plain water
Optional: add 2-3 drops of lavender essential oil or rose oil for fragrance

1. Mix the dry milk powder with just enough water to make a paste.

2. Gently massage the paste into your hair.

3. Cover hair with a hot towel for half an hour, changing the towel when it cools.

4. Rinse, shampoo, and end with your conditioner.

Products *Préférés*

Malheureusement, there comes a time when every glorious salon session comes to an end and we all have to maintain our stylist's genius work on our own. In order to do just that, French women pay close attention to the health of their hair and stock up on masks, treatments, and oils. Weekly deep treatments help keep their locks clean without having to wash again for another three to four days.

HMM, LESS FREQUENT WASHING WITHOUT SKIMPING ON A CLEAN LOOK? WE COULD GET BEHIND THAT IDEA!

When shampoo days do roll around, French women often opt for a non-lathering shampoo, and sometimes choose a mask instead of a conditioner. At this point, it should probably come as no surprise that they also adore soft, touchable locks and avoid using too many styling products so their hair doesn't get that cringe-worthy crunchy, stiff feeling. "They are looking for products that have nourishing properties," Greyl says.

TRÈS CHIC TRESSES: PRODUCTS TO HELP YOU RULE THE PARISIAN HAIR GAME

Want hair that's naturally cover-worthy, no glam squad required? Simplify your routine, banish heavy styling products, and stock up on these Parisian hair staples stat.

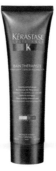

1.

NON-LATHERING SHAMPOO

Kérastase Paris Résistance Bain Thérapiste

2.

MASK

Christophe Robin Cleansing Mask With Lemon

3.

STYLING PRODUCT

Leonor Greyl Mousse au Lotus Volumatrice

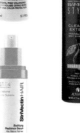

5.

DRY SHAMPOO

Alterna Haircare Cleanse Extend Translucent Dry Shampoo in Sugar Lemon

4.

TREATMENT

StriVectin® Hair Max Volume Bodifying Radiance Serum

The *Classique* French Style

When they're at the salon, French women definitely don't shy away from a daring new 'do if they're feeling it, but in general, they stick to naturally chic styles that don't look overdone. And they don't spend their free time at the blowout bar, either.

Want in on their mane moves? There are a few classically Parisian looks that are sure to get you *cheveux chics* in no time. "Try a haircut such as a classic bob (and not longer in the front!) or cut a strong fringe to your already long hair," Dimachki recommends.

WHATEVER CUT YOU DECIDE ON, CONSIDER YOUR LIFESTYLE AND THE HAIR YOU'RE ALREADY ROCKING, AND STEER CLEAR OF ANY 'DOS THAT VEER OFF THE FLATTERING PATH.

"Don't fight your natural texture and stick to colors that enhance your natural beauty," Peck says.

4 PARISIAN HAIR RULES TO LIVE BY

1. LET YOUR NATURAL HAIR SHINE THROUGH

How to: Air drying is so much better for your precious locks than damaging hot tools like flat irons and blow dryers, so lay off the constant barrage of hot air and usher your natural locks into the spotlight.

2. KEEP YOUR ROUTINE LOW-KEY

How to: Frequent trips to the salon and daily shampooing are so yesterday for *en vogue* French women, so cut down the time you dedicate to your hair care routine, because a busy gal like you doesn't have time to waste.

3. TOSS STICKY STYLING PRODUCTS ASIDE

How to: Layering on the gunky styling products means you need to shampoo more often, so steer clear of heavy products in favor of lighter hair stylers, and you'll be on the road to a *laissez-faire* routine.

4. COLOR SPARINGLY AND STRATEGICALLY

How to: Keep an eye out for hair colors that complement your skin tone and stay away from high maintenance hues that require lots of upkeep. After all, who wants to spend all that free time at the salon?

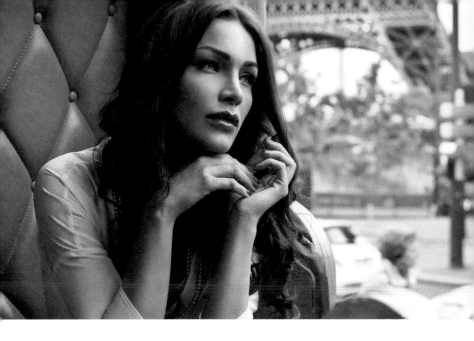

Nailing The Parisian Manicure

Manis and pedis are a guilty pleasure for many American women and we love frequent trips to the local nail salon, but Parisian women aren't as obsessed with nail care. Sure, they indulge in the occasional nail service and consider clean, well-groomed nails a beauty priority, but in the hierarchy of beauty importance, nails always fall behind skincare or waxing for *les Parisiennes*.

In other words, Parisian ladies are much more concerned with the state of their skin than the color of their tips on any given day. And they certainly don't stress about their nails enough to make any special effort to manicure them for a night out. "In the United States, a woman wouldn't dare go to an event (anything from a dinner to a black tie wedding) without nail polish. In France, it just wouldn't even be a top priority to make sure your nails were done," explains Jillian Babbitt, an American publicist who previously lived in Paris.

Pretty convenient, too, considering the fact that nail salons are few and far between in the city of Paris. To be honest, you're more likely to find a *boulangerie* or *pâtisserie* than you are a nail salon, and when you do stumble upon one, the prices are bound to be a bit high (supply and demand, *ma chérie*). "When I first moved to Paris and tried to find my local corner nail salon, I was in for a bit of a surprise! There were four bakeries on every corner but not a nail salon in sight! I quickly came to learn that this was not the norm for French women," Babbitt recalls.

Fuss-free nail routines mean most Parisians take care of their basic nail care at home, and many women let their nails go *sans couleur*. When they do reach for the polish bottle, Parisians keep it simple, and considering their subdued taste in makeup, it's not surprising that bold nail art, extreme nail polish shades, and long fake nails don't exactly tickle their fancy. Instead, these ladies prefer a subtle approach and flock towards natural colors, delicate hues, and classic reds (like their favorite lipsticks!).

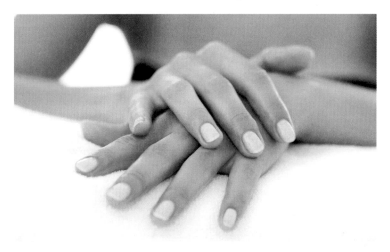

Traditional French Hand Bath

Soon you'll have super-smooth hands with glossy nails and not a dark spot in sight!

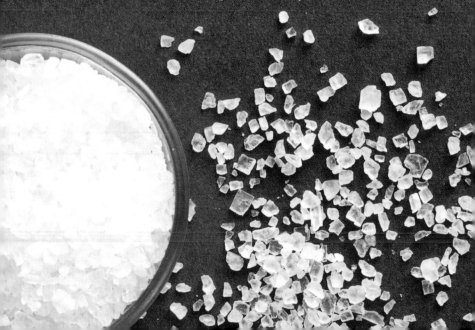

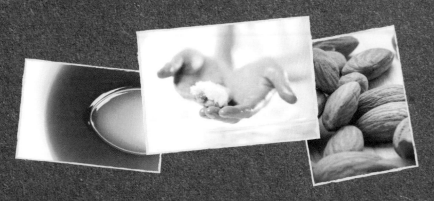

What Makes It Parisian?

Those chic Parisian women don't believe in covering their hands with ultra-opaque nail polish or humongous cocktail rings. Hence, they need flawless skin and nails.

What Does It Do?

The salt rids the hands of dead skin; while the olive and almond oils provide a hefty dose of hydration.

Ingredients

2 tablespoons coarse sea salt granules
1 tablespoon virgin olive oil
2-3 drops of almond oil

1. Pour the salt into a bowl.

2. Add the olive oil.

3. Scoop out a handful of the mixture in your palms and scrub your hands thoroughly.

4. Rinse hands with warm water and dab some almond oil on the nails.

GARLIC FOR NAILS

Garlic strengthens nails and helps them grow longer. And the strong smell disappears in about half an hour!

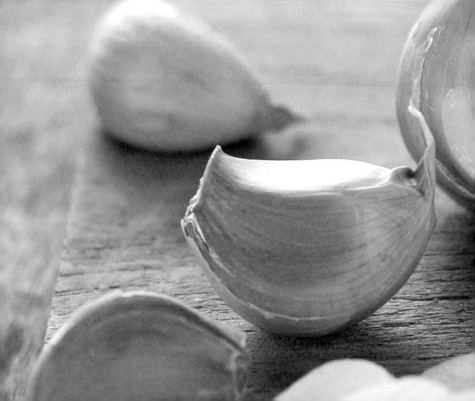

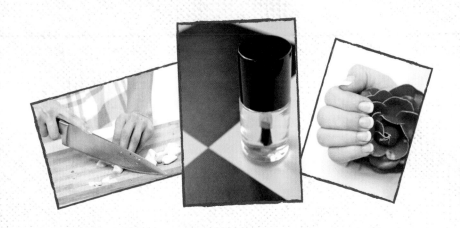

What Makes It Parisian?

Garlic, a staple in Parisian cuisine, is about as French as a vegetable can get.

What Does it Do?

Garlic strengthens the nails and helps them grow longer and stronger.

Ingredients

¼ teaspoon of fresh garlic, finely chopped
A bottle of clear nail polish

1. Add the garlic to the bottle of clear nail polish.

2. Let the bottle sit in a cool, dry place for a week.

3. Use this concoction as a clear or base coat whenever you polish your nails.

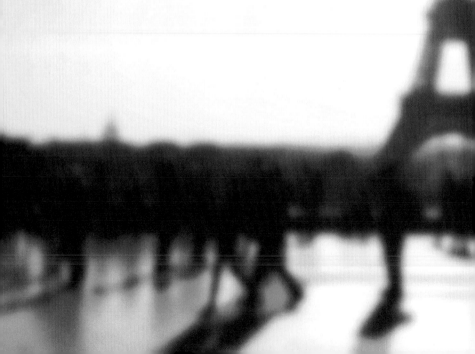

PARISIAN STYLE:

The Art of Looking Effortlessly Chic

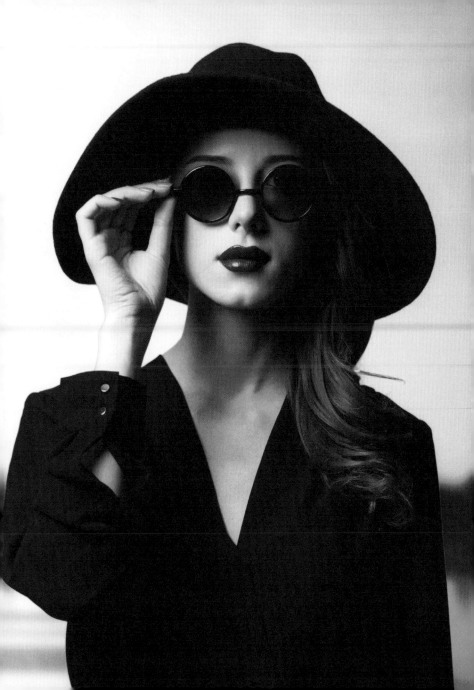

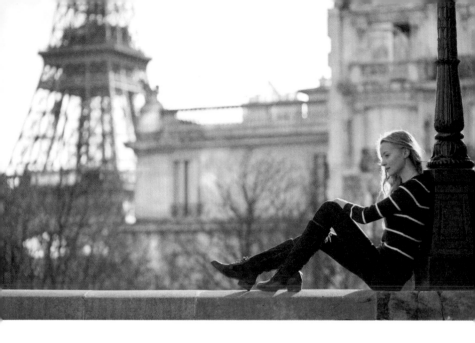

Immaculately tied scarves. Cute little flats that never seem to quit. And impeccably tailored wardrobe essentials that suit a woman's personal style to a T. Yep, Parisian women definitely have that style *je ne sais quoi* perfected! So much so that it's safe to say at some point, we've all coveted their sartorial sense. It just so happens we've personally never stopped admiring Parisians' flair for *la mode* and we don't think we will anytime soon.

French women take a certain pride in their appearance, yet they seem to look chic without trying at all. It's that relaxed attitude that makes us all jealous and totally adoring at the same time.

So are all French women born fluent in fashion or is it something in the water of the Seine? All kidding aside, we've often wondered whether *les Parisiennes* are blessed with a knack for style or if living in such a *très chic* city rubs off on them. Perhaps it's a little bit of both!

"The style of French women is definitely something that is in our culture and passed down from generation to generation. Yes, France is known for their fashion houses and '*je ne sais quoi*,' but really the essence of personal style for any French woman is taking the historic fashion influence our culture is known for and adapting it to her lifestyle," says New York City-based French shoe designer Jean-Michel Cazabat.

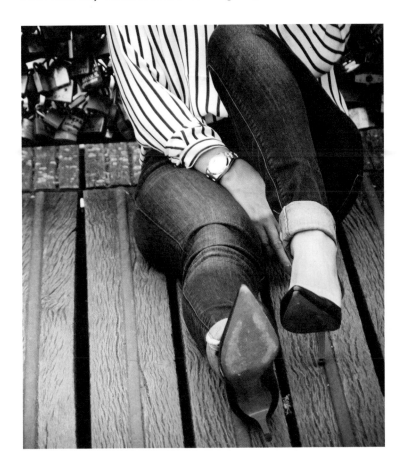

THE MODERN PARISIAN FASHIONISTA CAN MERGE *HAUTE COUTURE* AND FAST FASHION, VINTAGE AND *NOUVEAU* BRANDS IN A TOTALLY ENVIABLE WAY THAT MAKES US ALL DROP OUR JAWS AND STARE. AND THAT'S PRETTY RAD.

The art of dressing seems to come pretty instinctually to them, too. So does that mean we can add a sixth sense (the sense of style) to the list of reasons why we love Parisian women? Well, that and the fact that they actually listen to their moms when it comes to fashion advice.

"I think for most Parisian women their first fashion inspiration was their mother. The first timeless and high-quality piece you own is usually given to you by your mother or is a piece you borrowed from

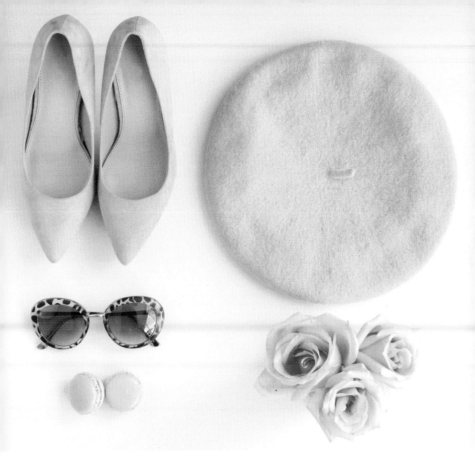

her closet!" says Camille Parruitte, Parisian founder of the jewelry line Nouvel Heritage. "When I was in high school, I remember borrowing my mother's cashmere sweaters and how they made me feel like a woman. Style, to some extent, is like family heritage. You internalize your mother's style and try to build your own with the basics she gave you."

Ok, so they fuse high and low style effortlessly *and* take fashion advice from their moms? We can definitely learn a thing or two about style from Parisian gals!

JASMINE POWDER

Use this finely textured, beautifully scented concoction as a dusting powder, deodorant, or to prevent chafing. Those Parisian women especially bring it out when they're going for the seductive kill!

What Makes It Parisian?

This powder represents the principles of jasmine *effleurage*, which has made the French town of Grasse the perfume capital of the world.

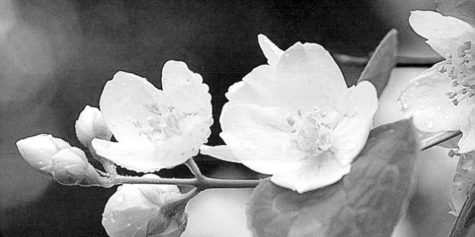

What Does It Do?

French chalk is what we know as talcum powder. It's perfect for absorbing excess oil and moisture, and for keeping skin soft, matte, cool, and dry. Jasmine is one of aromatherapy's most popular scents and has a soothing, and revitalizing effect. It's also one of nature's most potent aphrodisiacs! Civet, ambergris, and white sugar candy help "fix" the scent, making it last longer.

Ingredients

French chalk
Fine sieve
Lidded box
Jasmine flowers
1-2 grains civet musk
1-2 grains ambergris
¼ teaspoon white sugar candy

1. Powder the French chalk if it's in solid form.

2. Sift the powder through a fine sieve.

3. Layer the sieved powder at the bottom of the box.

4. Pour the jasmine flowers on the powder; close the lid and let stand in a cool, dry place.

5. Change flowers every 24 hours until powder is well impregnated with the jasmine scent. Then throw away all the petals.

6. Rub together the civet, ambergris, and white sugar candy and mix them with the powder.

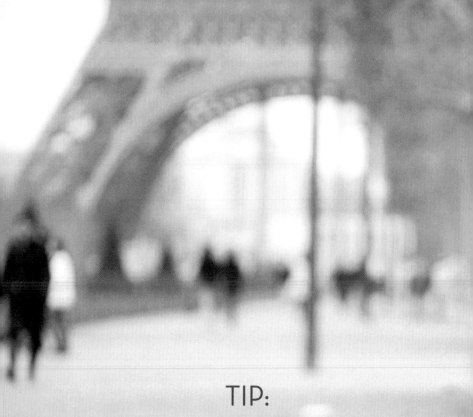

TIP:
The essence of personal style
for any French woman is taking
the historic fashion influence
our culture is known for and
adapting it to her lifestyle!

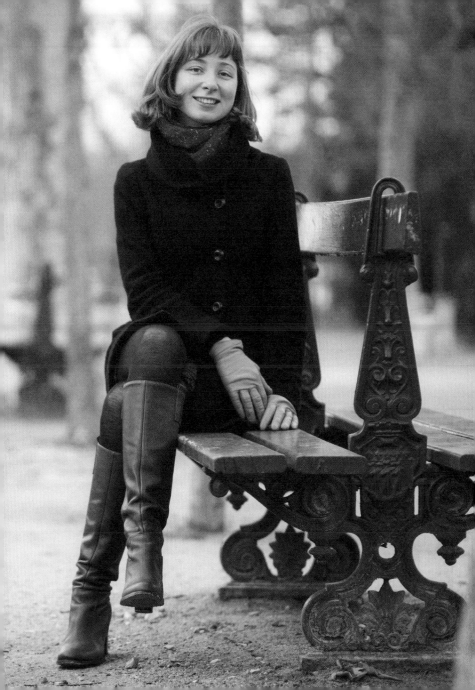

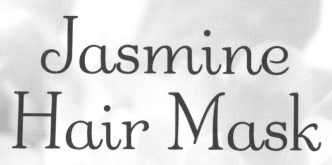

Jasmine Hair Mask

The beautiful, exotic scent of jasmine will linger in your hair long after the mask is washed away.

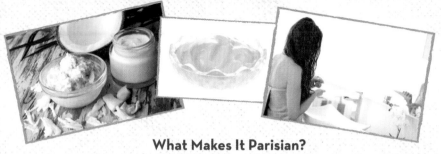

What Makes It Parisian?

French women would rather take care of the basics—like the health of their hair—than resort to measures such as complicated blow dries and chemical-laden styling products.

What Does It Do?

This hair mask will relax and purify the scalp, along with stimulating blood circulation and encouraging hair growth. It's also a great nourisher for dry and frizzy strands, turning them smooth, sleek, and glossy with regular use.

Ingredients

1 cup fresh jasmine flowers
1 cup yogurt
1 tablespoon coconut oil

1. Crush the jasmine flowers to release the oils.

2. Add the yogurt and coconut oil; and mix well.

3. Apply this paste to dry hair, pre-shampoo.

4. Put on a tight bathing cap (or wrap your head with plastic film) and cover with a hot towel; let this remain for half an hour, then shampoo as usual.

STYLE EXPERTS' TIPS FOR AN *EN VOGUE* FRENCH LOOK

In the market for an *à la mode* look? Consider these 6 expert fashion tips your passport to Parisian style.

1. "When in doubt, buy a few timeless and high-quality pieces."

-- CAMILLE PARRUITTE, PARISIAN FOUNDER OF THE JEWELRY LINE NOUVEL HERITAGE

2. "Mix classics with color and fun statement pieces."

-- JENNIFER CUVILLIER, STYLE DIRECTOR OF PARIS' FAMOUS DEPARTMENT STORE LE BON MARCHÉ

3. "Less is more: It's a common saying in fashion, but one I think French women abide by."

-- NEW YORK CITY-BASED FRENCH SHOE DESIGNER JEAN-MICHEL CAZABAT

4. "Wear clothes that both make you feel comfortable and are comfortable."

-- CAMILLE PARRUITTE

5. "Do not follow every trend."

-- JENNIFER CUVILLIER

6. "Have fun with accessories: Shoes, bags, jewelry, and scarfs are all fun and easy ways to bring color and fun into your wardrobe."

-- JEAN-MICHEL CAZABAT

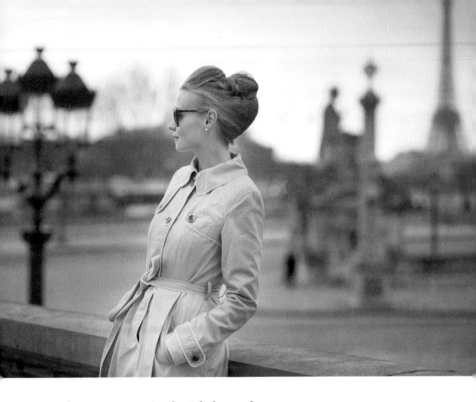

The Parisian Style *Philosophie*

Before you begin the fun part—you know, building your wardrobe and a little thing called shopping!—understanding the philosophy behind Parisian style is key to adapting it to your own American lifestyle.

Les Parisiennes have a natural instinct for personal style and a cool inner confidence that helps them rock classic and trendy looks alike. And that last part is pretty essential if you ask Jennifer Cuvillier, style director of Paris' famous department store Le Bon Marché: "The French style is all about how you wear and put your clothes together. It's an attitude, an intellectual art of dressing."

Part of that confidence, of course, is knowing just how much effort to put into your outfit without looking like a fashion wannabe.

"Your style is part of your identity and is what gives the first impression when you meet someone," Parruitte reveals. "Yet, style is not something you need to put a lot of work into; it should be natural. When it comes to choosing your style, you need to trust your instinct and wear what you like best."

Naturally, we all want to take our style to the next level with a few finishing touches and tiny details, but Parisians' conscientious effort always flies under the radar. "A French woman always looks put together, but never in an obvious way. The details are subtle and the silhouette is always pretty and feminine but with an organic approach," Cazabat explains.

Now that you've got a clear grasp on the Parisian style *je ne sais quoi*, the next step in your quest for looking effortlessly chic like a Parisian is tackling your wardrobe!

10 FASHION STAPLES FOR A *CLASSIQUE* FRENCH LOOK

Dying to perfect your Parisian style know-how? Mix and match these 10 wardrobe staples with your own trendy and timeless gems, and you'll be on the road to French fashion fame.

1. Cashmere sweater
2. White blouse
3. Slim jeans
4. Little black dress
5. Moto jacket
6. Breton shirt
7. Trench jacket
8. Lace lingerie
9. Fitted blazer
10. Silk blouse

French Wardrobe *Essentiels*

Want to look the part of a stylish French woman? Step in line, sister! And get ready to curate a wardrobe mixed with timeless and trendy pieces that scream *très chic*.

It's no secret that Parisians have a penchant for the color black (and all neutral shades, for that matter!), and their love affair with the more subdued colors in life actually serves a quite useful fashion purpose.

"These colors are the must purchased and worn the most often because they can be matched and paired with most anything. They are timeless and can be dressed up or down depending on the occasion," Cuvillier explains.

LESSON LEARNED: THE FIRST STEP TO BUILDING YOUR PARISIAN WARDROBE IS TO THINK NEUTRAL!

Bien sûr, that doesn't mean you can't have fun with trendy and classic prints alike and bold color — in fact, it's encouraged.

"In Paris you do see pops of color and prints. Red is always a festive color to wear, leopard is a fun print to play with, and color blocking in recent years has also helped incorporate pops of color into one's wardrobe," Cuvillier says. But Parisian women understand that a subtle statement sometimes goes the furthest distance, and they make a point to invest in neutral basics they can mix and match with their bolder hues.

They also know a thing or two about accessorizing. Sumptuous silk scarves, fashionable flats, delicate touches of jewelry, *de rigueur* black pumps, and a classic handbag that goes with everything are all *nécessaire* items to add to your shopping list! And when used in moderation, they make a *grand* impact.

LESSON NUMBER TWO? STOCK UP ON SUBTLY CHIC ACCESSORIES BUT LEAVE OVER-ACCESSORIZING FOR THE AMATEURS.

Parisian style staples like cashmere sweaters, slim jeans, a crisp white blouse, a little black dress, a super cool leather jacket, striped Breton shirts, lace lingerie, a fitted blazer, and a tailored coat will get a lot of mileage in your closet because you can mix and match them with just about anything. And that takes us to lesson number three:

INVEST IN TIMELESS WARDROBE STAPLES YOU'LL ADORE FOR YEARS TO COME AND THAT WILL NEVER GO OUT OF STYLE.

While you're packing your closet with must-have essentials, don't leave out one easily forgotten detail: tailoring. Flattering silhouettes and top-notch tailoring are a surefire way to make your clothes look *très cher* and Parisians hold the figure-flattering practice near and dear.

"The tailored look is very Parisian. It stems back to the origins of the first fashion houses in Paris — the streamlined skirts, fitted jackets, and overall feminine aesthetic. Parisian women purchase key pieces with the intent to wear them over a long period of time, so the fit is key," Cuvillier says. "If you are investing in a piece, why not take the extra step to ensure it fits you properly? Tailoring should be a universal tool for all women. It can really transform any look."

Smart thinking, right? Now once you've got your wardrobe ready, it's time to take your new purchases out for a test drive!

NEUTRAL IN *NOIR*

Parisians have an undeniable *amour* for the color black, and when all-black outfits look this gosh darn classy, we really can't fault them. Join in on their *noir* know-how with these fashion finds.

1. Modcloth Rhyme or Parisian Sweater

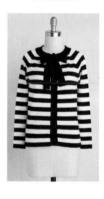

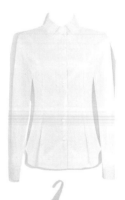

2. Anne Fontaine "Larry" Blouse in Stretch Poplin with Long Sleeves and a Single-Cuff

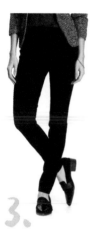

3. Old Navy The Long Pixie Pants in Black Jack 3

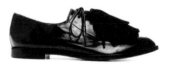

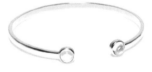

4. Wren + Glory Stone Cuff

5. Loeffler Randall Jasper in Black

LADY IN *ROUGE*

Wine tastes great, but it also looks pretty darn amazing as a dress color. Worn with a timeless tweed jacket, stylish black pumps, and a cool bag, this style will have you looking like a Bordeaux babe.

1.

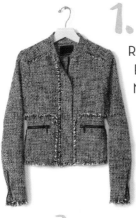

Banana Republic Raw-Edge Tweed Moto Jacket

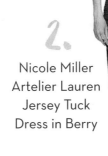

2.

Nicole Miller Artelier Lauren Jersey Tuck Dress in Berry

3.

Ghurka Doyenne Mini in Charcoal

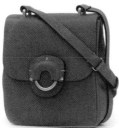

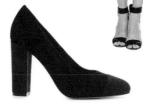

4. Jean-Michel Cazabat Glitter Blocked Heel

TRENCH CHIC

Every Parisian fashionista needs a trench coat,
a *fabuleux* scarf (or 10!), a striped Breton top, a pair of
jeans, and some neutral flats. They're all style essentials
you can mix and match with other items, or throw
together for a flawless look in five minutes or less.

1.

Small Trades Classic
Striped ¾ Sleeve
T-Shirt, available
at Zady.com

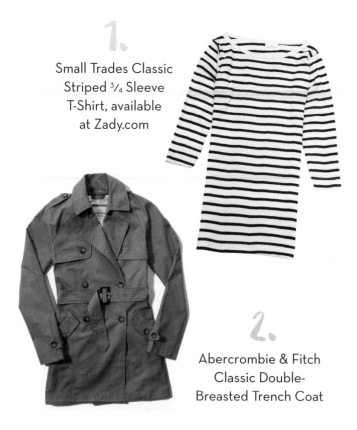

2.

Abercrombie & Fitch
Classic Double-
Breasted Trench Coat

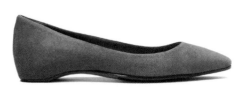

3.

Aquatalia
Marcella Flat
in Caramel

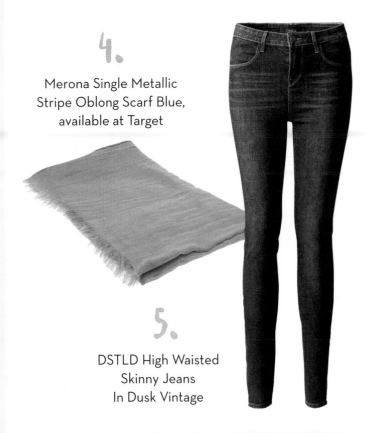

4.

Merona Single Metallic
Stripe Oblong Scarf Blue,
available at Target

5.

DSTLD High Waisted
Skinny Jeans
In Dusk Vintage

Dress Like a *Parisienne*

So you're ready to walk the chic walk and dress like a Parisian, huh? *Impecc!* Make sure you're armed with some useful tips to store in your perfectly tailored back pocket.

First things first, Parisian women approach style in a similar way as they do makeup: with a soft touch.

WHEN IT COMES TO THE ART OF DRESSING, REMEMBER THAT LESS IS ALWAYS MORE, SO TRY NOT TO TRY SO HARD.

No, try a bit less. Wait, are you confused yet? Okay, good because the whole allure of a French woman's style is to keep you guessing on just how much effort she put into her look.

The classic Parisian fashionista wants to look effortlessly chic, yet never overdone. And she knows how to mix timeless basics with trendy pieces like it's nobody's business. So sneakers and a little black dress? Yep, they'll rock that look. Designer blazers with vintage T-shirts? Totally on their fashion radar.

The key is knowing there's a time and a place for everything, and every outfit. "We emphasize that every occasion has its proper

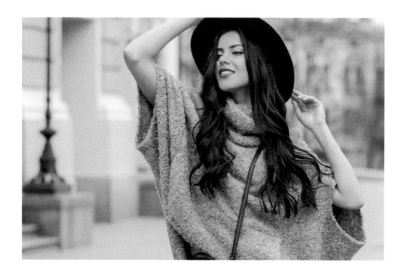

dressing code, and you would not dress the same to go to the office as you would to go to dinner outside," Parruitte explains.

That means you sometimes have to reinvent the items you've already got hanging in your closet! So make sure you build a strong, versatile wardrobe with timeless staples you can mix and match in *beaucoup* ways!

And don't be afraid to have fun with some impulse fast fashion purchases every now and again. "I believe Parisian women are more concerned with quality than quantity, and therefore they will use fast fashion to complete their wardrobe," Parruitte says.

Trends are fun and all, but French women are no slaves to style when it comes to following the latest runway looks. Personal style and under-stated elegance are far more important to them than blending into the trendy crowd, so Parisians put a lot of effort into looking effortless.

One genius way they do just that? Through the subtle use of accessories.

5 MUST-HAVE ACCESSORIES FOR TIMELESS PARISIAN STYLE

One of the best-kept secrets of French style? Their keen ability to accessorize in just the right way. A pair of flats here, a silk scarf there – they all add a certain flair that makes everyone do a double take. Want in on their accessorizing act? Head to a chic boutique and stock up on these five must-have accessories for a uniquely Parisian look.

1.

FRAGRANCE

Because everyone knows that fragrance is an absolutely essential accessory for Parisian women.

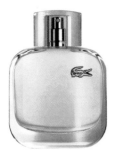

Lacoste L.12.12 Pour Elle Natural 1.6 OZ Spray

2.

SCARF

The best *part* about a *classique* scarf? You can tie it a different way every day of the week!

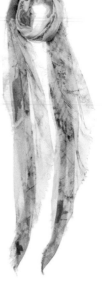

Mangrove "Bittersweet" Scarf in Purple

3. FLATS

Parisian women are always on the go, so they need cute flats that can keep up with their mobile lifestyle.

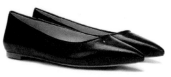

Original Collection by Dr. Scholl's Shoes Tenacious Flat in Black Leather

4. CLASSIC BAG

Trends come and go, but a classic structured bag will always be *en vogue* for the ever chic French woman.

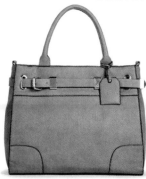

JustFab Mario Bag in Mauve

5. DELICATE JEWELRY

Jewelry is subtle and personal for our Parisian friends, who prefer delicate pieces and classic styles (like pearls!) over trendy baubles.

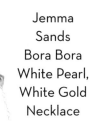

Jemma Sands Bora Bora White Pearl, White Gold Necklace

A *Femme* and Her Accessories

As a shoe designer, Cazabat knows a thing or two about *les chaussures*, and he says French women keep an open mind when choosing the stylish accessories that adorn their feet. But they do err on the side of practicality when it comes to heel height. "French women, like most women, love all types of shoes. They especially love shoes with clean lines and classic silhouettes," he says. "French women also do not wear very tall heels like American women; they prefer smaller heels and flats."

Yet another reason to love these stylish gals. Parisian women love to walk all over the city (wouldn't you if you lived in the world's most gorgeous place?), so guess you could say Parisian ladies' shoes of choice were made for walking!

Lucky for us, flats are comfy and cute, and you can dress them up or down. So if you're looking for a simple way to add an instant touch of Parisian flair to your look, just swap your go-to heels for a versatile pair of loafers, a classic pair of oxfords, or a girly pair of ballet flats! They'll pair well with pants, skirts, and dresses alike, so the options are endless.

Typically, we women are, shall we say, collectors of footwear. But for ladies in Paris, the focus is more on the make of *les chaussures*, and a bit less on their growing collection. "Parisian women prefer quality vs. quantity. They value good leather, craftsmanship, and design," Cazabat explains.

But their affair with accessories doesn't stop there. Parisian women also love jewelry and when it comes to their *bijoux*, it's all about pieces with character and history, not flashy, oversized baubles.

"I think French woman have a very personal connection with their jewelry. They love small and dainty pieces," jewelry designer

Parruitte describes. "But most importantly, they love the stories behind their jewelry. We love pieces that were given to us by loved ones. The most precious ones would probably come from your parents or grandparents."

For an authentic French look, steer clear of heavy jewelry layering and swap some of those oversize costume-y pieces we all adore so much in favor of some delicate pendants and bracelets.

And while you're accessorizing, don't forget the most important Parisian accessory of all: fragrance.

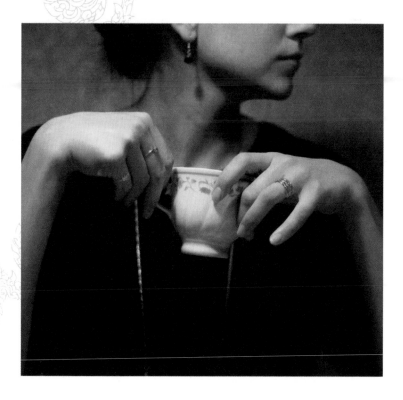

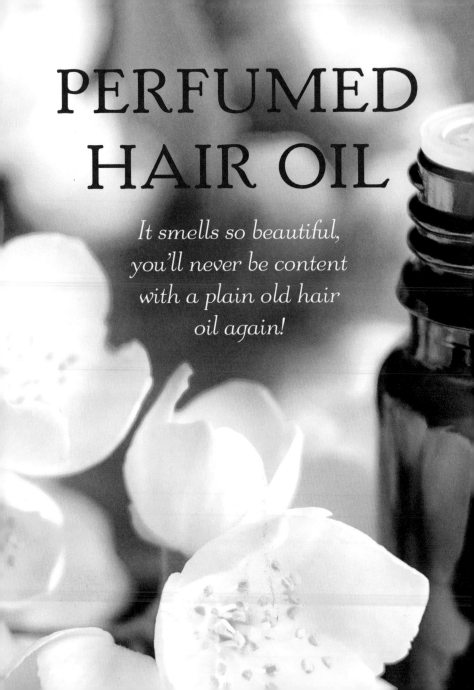

PERFUMED HAIR OIL

It smells so beautiful, you'll never be content with a plain old hair oil again!

What Makes It Parisian?

Parisian women love products that can multitask: in this case, a hefty dose of fragrant aromatherapy combined with hair-boosting goodness.

What Does It Do?

Rose and jasmine are both known for their mood-boosting, stress relieving, and aphrodisiacal benefits!

Ingredients

2 cups tuberose or jasmine flowers
6 cups olive oil or sweet almond oil
Mortar & pestle
Lidded glass jar
Strainer or cheesecloth

1. Gently bruise the flowers with the mortar and pestle (or a blunt object).

2. Pour the flowers into the glass jar.

3. Add the oil; lid the jar and let it stand in the sun for 15 days.

4. Strain out the flowers and squeeze them to draw out all remaining oil; add this oil back to the jar.

5. Repeat the whole process at least 3 times to truly impregnate the oil with the fragrance of the flowers.

6. When the aroma has reached your desired potency, filter out all the flowers and store the liquid in a tightly capped glass bottle.

Rose Petal Lip Balm

This pretty-smelling lip balm feels unbelievably emollient and just sinks into the lips, leaving a soft, rosy flush. You can even use it for your hands and nipples.

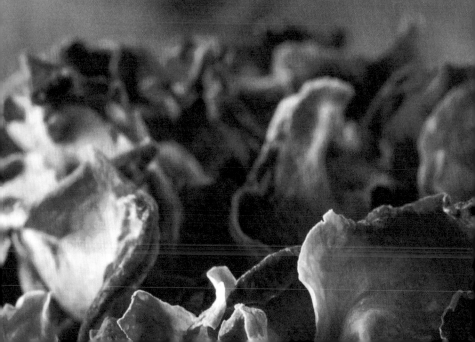

What Makes It Parisian?

A red lip is the French makeup signature and we all know lipstick doesn't sit well on dry or chapped lips. Hence, French women take their lip care very seriously, especially when it involves roses.

What Does It Do?

The beeswax and sweet almond oil preserve lips' fragile tissue. Roses contain high levels of vitamin C, oils, and proteins, which help keep skin soft and moisturized. Plus, they are high in retinol (vitamin A), which treats lines, wrinkles, and other visible signs of aging.

Ingredients

2½ ounces beeswax, grated
¼ pint sweet almond oil
3 tablespoons dried rose petals

1. Gently crush the rose petals to release the natural oils.

2. Add the petals to the almond oil.

3. Gently warm the oil over low heat for a couple of minutes (it shouldn't boil).

4. Remove the oil; cover and leave to infuse overnight.

5. Put the infusion back on low heat and add the beeswax.

6. Stir until everything melts and is well blended.

7. Strain out the rose petals.

8. Pour the mixture into small tin or glass boxes; let solidify a bit and then use daily.

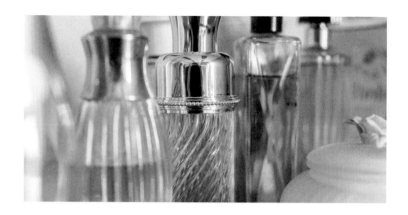

Parfum, the Essential Parisian Accessory

You might be tempted to group fragrance into the beauty category (and most people do!), but for Parisian women, it's an essential style accessory. No outfit is complete without perfume, and it adds a touch of attitude, complementing your ensemble as much as any other accessory.

But perfume isn't just some other mindless accessory for Parisian women; to them, it's a revered ritual with great cultural significance. And it's no longer just a luxury item reserved for the upper class, like it once was; these days, perfume is ubiquitous. "Since the 2000s it has become more affordable, and French women apply it to finish their look and as a seduction tool. It is considered to be very refined," says Leonor Greyl president Caroline Greyl.

Parisiennes take style inspiration from their moms, and they also consider them to be fragrance muses. "Beauty products and our beauty routines oftentimes stem from our mothers. Watching them getting ready and admiring all of their products and perfume as a child has an influence on one's personal taste as they grow up," reveals Elisabeth Holder, co-president of Ladurée US.

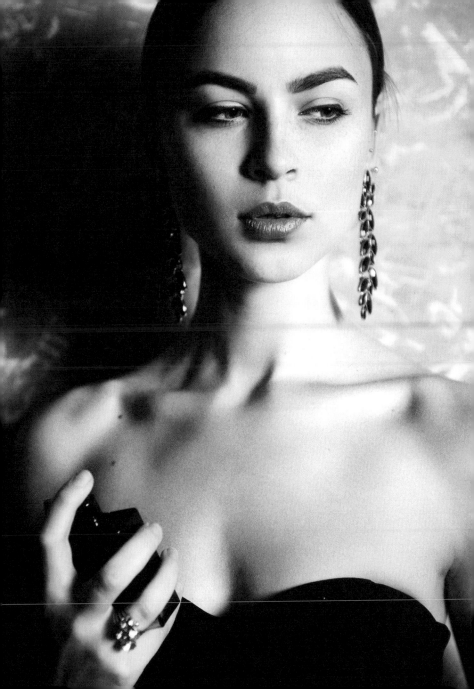

FRENCH MILLED SOAP

French milling creates the smoothest, most luxurious bar of soap in the world. No self-respecting Parisian would go for anything less!

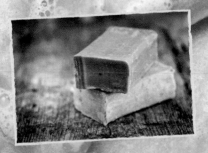

What Makes It Parisian?
This is an ancient soap making technique discovered by French soap makers in the 1700s.

What Does It Do?
Milling extracts excess water from the soap. This not only creates a longer lasting product but also ensures that the ingredients are well blended and that the soap bar's texture is smoother and more uniform, *sans* impurities.

Ingredients

3 bars any unscented natural soap
1 cup warm water or coconut milk
Additives (choose from aromatic essential oils,
herbs, colloidal oatmeal, flower petals etc.)
Cheese grater
Double boiler or non-reactive pot
Wooden spoon
Soap molds
Wax paper

1. Grate soap bars into a double boiler or non-reactive pot, then add water or coconut milk; mix well.

2. Heat on low, stirring often with a wooden spoon. If bubbles form, stop stirring until they cease; if soap starts drying out, add more water or coconut milk.

3. When soap flakes melt, remove mixture from the heat and add additives (except essential oils).

4. Stir mixture until it's cool but pourable, then add oils.

5. Spoon mixture into molds, packing well to avoid air bubbles. Once molds are full, tap gently against counter to settle soap and remove air pockets; then set aside to dry.

6. Once hard, remove soap from molds and set on wax paper in a cool, dark place to cure thoroughly (this may take a few weeks).

7. Turn soaps once weekly; they're ready when you can press them with your finger and not leave an impression.

8. Wrap soaps in fun paper of your choice to gift or store!

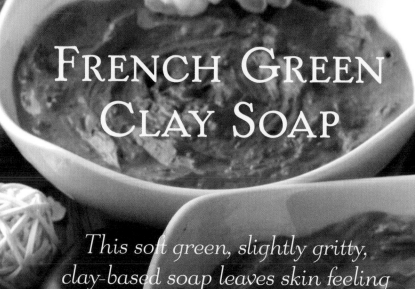

FRENCH GREEN CLAY SOAP

This soft green, slightly gritty, clay-based soap leaves skin feeling super-clean. It's also particularly good for acne.

What Makes It Parisian?
Green clay, which comes from the quarries in France, is a staple in soaps from the region.

What Does It Do?
Made of mineral-rich volcanic ash, green clay's molecular structure helps it pull out deeply seated toxins and balance skin's pH levels.

Ingredients
2 bars any olive oil-based soap
1 teaspoon green clay
$\frac{1}{2}$ to 1 teaspoon any aromatic essential oil
1 tablespoon fine sea salt
1 cup warm water
Double boiler
Soap molds (you can use cookie cutters)

1. Melt soap bars in the double boiler on medium heat; avoid letting the liquid boil.

2. Lower heat to a slow simmer. Add green clay and mix well. Add essential oil and mix again.

3. Pour mixture into molds, leaving an inch at the top; let cool and harden.

4. Once hardened, remove from the molds; cut into desired shape or size using a sharp knife, if necessary.

5. Combine sea salt with warm water and wash soap bars in this solution. Let soap dry completely, then rinse in plain warm water.

6. Wrap the bars in fun, Paris-inspired paper to store (or gift)!

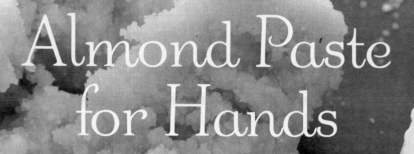

Almond Paste
for Hands

This paste feels slightly coarse and you will need to really massage it into the skin – but it's all worth the effort for perfectly smooth hands.

What Makes It Parisian?

Almonds from the South of France have long been revered the world over for their skin-nourishing properties and robust scent.

What Does It Do?

Almonds are *très* rich in calcium and minerals and leave skin soft and smooth.

Ingredients

1 cup bitter almonds
3 cups whole milk
4-5 white bread crumbs
Mortar & pestle (or food processor, set on low)
Heavy bottomed kettle

1. Blanch almonds in warm water and remove skins. Leave almonds to dry out completely.

2. Beat the almonds in the mortar or food processor, adding just enough milk to form a paste.

3. Soak bread crumbs in milk and add them to the almonds; beat together until everything is well mixed. Pour this mixture into the kettle.

4. Add enough milk to completely cover the mixture and let simmer over low heat until it turns to the texture of a soft paste; keep adding more milk if the mixture starts to look dry.

5. Scoop paste into a glass bottle and store in the fridge.

6 *POPULAIRE* SHOPPING HOT SPOTS IN PARIS

If shopping is high on your priority list when you visit Paris (*bien sûr*), you'll be in paradise. From *charmant* boutiques to massive department stores, the city is filled with options galore, and these noteworthy gems are definitely worth a stop on your next visit to the City of Light.

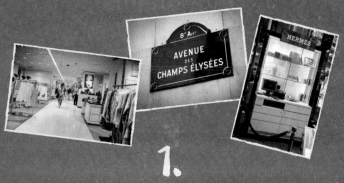

1.

GALERIES LAFAYETTE:

Paris' 9th arrondissement is home to this beloved department store where only the breathtaking view from the roof surpasses the amazing assortment of clothes.

2.

CHAMPS ÉLYSÉES:

No trip to Paris is complete without a jaunt down the city's most famous fashion avenue filled with a myriad of luxury shops. The street even has a song named after it!

3.
LE BON MARCHÉ:

It's almost as fun strolling around admiring the cool artwork and fun window displays in this department store as it is browsing through its clothing selection. Almost!

4.
PRINTEMPS:

Add this architectural wonder, founded in 1865, to your list of must-see Paris buildings. The best part? Admission is free. But we can't promise you'll walk away without spending anything.

5.
RUE SAINT-HONORÉ:

Bring one (or two) of your best cards with you if you're planning to do some damage on this luxury shopping street. You only live once, right?

6.
MONOPRIX:

Find fashion, home goods, food, and more at this one-stop shop with multiple locations throughout Paris.

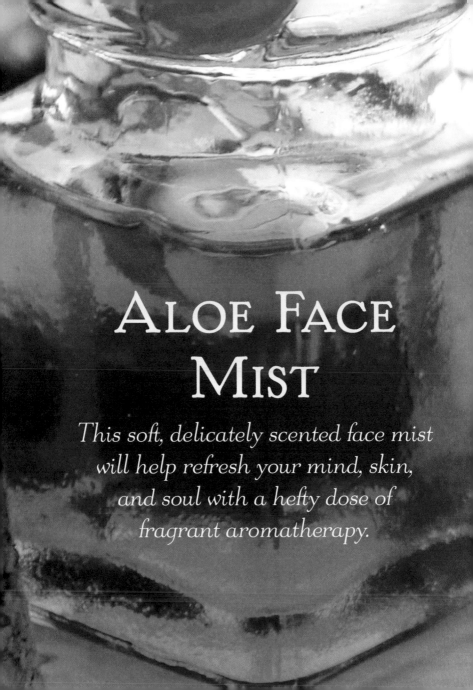

ALOE FACE MIST

This soft, delicately scented face mist will help refresh your mind, skin, and soul with a hefty dose of fragrant aromatherapy.

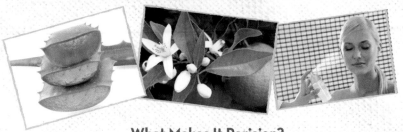

What Makes It Parisian?

Unlike most others, Parisian women don't shun the sun. Instead, they venture out confident in their ability to defend themselves against its damaging properties, while still soaking in its goodness.

What Does It Do?

Orange blossom water calms and tones with its gentle astringency, lavender essential oil helps reduce inflammation, and aloe vera moisturizes and encourages skin's healing abilities.

Ingredients

½ cup aloe vera juice
½ cup orange blossom water
3 drops lavender essential oil
A spray bottle

1. Fill a small spray bottle halfway with aloe vera juice.

2. Add enough orange blossom water to nearly fill the bottle to the top.

3. Add 3 drops of lavender essential oil; shake well.

4. Shake again before every use.

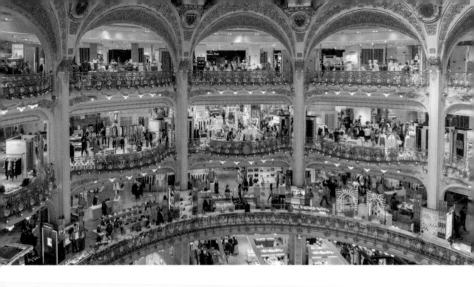

Shop Like a Parisian: The Art of *"Les Soldes"*

Sure we love Paris for its culture, its gorgeous architecture, and its *délicieux* food, but let's be honest, we've also got quite a soft spot for the incredible shopping in the City of Light. From the fashion-filled Champs-Élysées to the famous Le Bon Marché and Galeries Lafayette, Paris is chock-full of tempting stores just waiting to whet your style appetite.

And if you play your cards right, you might just score some pretty sweet deals if you visit the city during its biannual *"les soldes."* These blink-and-you'll-miss-them sales only happen twice a year for a few weeks at a time (winter and summer) and draw huge crowds of native Parisians and tourists alike, so you better get ready for some competition while you're out hunting for bargains!

But don't get too seduced by the draw of a sale sticker, ladies. The key to French style is knowing what works for your body and your personal style, right? So you can actually learn a thing or two from *les soldes* on how to avoid getting caught up in the whirlwind of a sale.

"Smart shopping is key, even if it's not during *les soldes*. It's about knowing your closet, what you actually need, and what pieces work for you," Cuvillier reveals.

IT'S ABOUT KNOWING WHAT PIECES WORK FOR YOU.

The bottom line? Head into any shopping trip—sale or not—with a mental list of what your key wardrobe staples are and what items you could actually use to jazz them up a bit. There's no use buying items that don't work for your body, your lifestyle, or your wardrobe, after all! Then head into the store ready to turn away any tempting items that don't fit that criteria, no matter how good the sale might be.

"A lot of women (both French and American) can sometimes get too excited with a sale and purchase items hastily," Cuvillier says. "My advice: Less splurge buying, and smart investment buying. You and your closet will thank you for it in the future."

Tackling the store with a friend or family member can sometimes lead to impulse purchases, but if you head into it telling them to keep you in check, they can actually keep you accountable! Shopping, after all, is more fun with *une amie*!

"I think that *les soldes* is also a social event," Parruitte says. "This is usually the time of the year you invite your girlfriends or mother/sisters to shop with you. A day of shopping is always more productive and entertaining when spent in good company!"

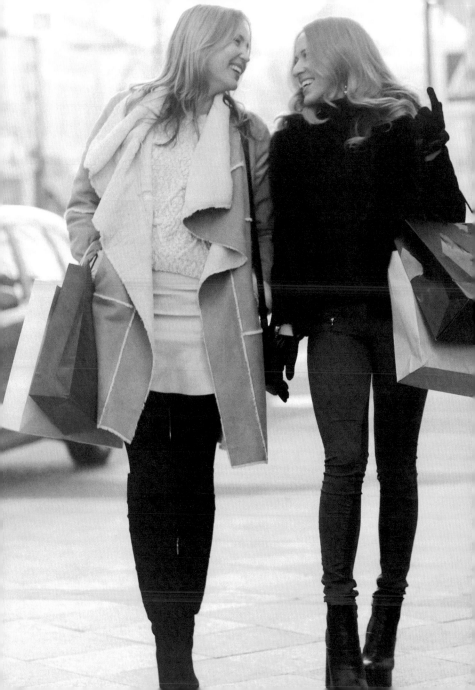

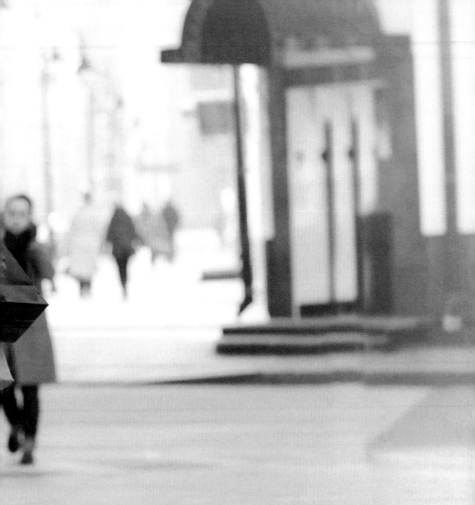

LA VIE EN PARIS:

Lifestyle and Self-Care Secrets

L eisurely strolls through Le Jardin de Luxembourg, generous lunch breaks, and a sweet work-life balance—yep, French women basically have this whole lifestyle thing mastered. The more time you spend in Paris, the more you start to appreciate the *très* laid-back culture and Parisians' carefully crafted approach to lifestyle. You see, *ma chérie*, life for the fashionable French *femme* is lived one stylish step at a time and features a well-balanced schedule filled with copious amounts of self-care.

French women work hard, but they also play and relax hard. And if you haven't come down with a major case of style or beauty envy for our Parisian *amies* just yet, prepare to soon because their work-life balance, sleeping habits, relaxing bath routine, and grooming habits are bound to make you turn green with envy.

Work-Life Balance, the *Européen* Way

Fine-tuning the perfect recipe for a work-life balance can sometimes seem like a massive task that's slightly out of your reach, but with a little trial and error, *c'est possible*!

Even though French women hardly "have it all," they certainly know a thing or two about the *laissez-faire* lifestyle we covet so much.

Take the typical French workweek, for instance. Our friends in France have enjoyed a 35-hour workweek for many years while most American women working full-time clock in at least 40 hours a week (before overtime). *Bien sûr*, a lot of French women put in a fair deal of overtime themselves, depending on their profession. But the point is, even if the standard 35-hour workweek changes (and rumors are it might), the French definitely have their workers' backs and keep their eyes on a work-life balance when it comes to the number of hours their employees work.

THE FRENCH DEFINITELY KEEP THEIR EYES ON A WORK-LIFE BALANCE.

If you weren't experiencing major *jalousie* yet, just wait *une minute*! Did you know Parisian women enjoy *beaucoup* vacation time compared to their American counterparts? Yep, and they're not afraid to take it either. In fact, if you've ever visited the city towards the end of the summer, you'll notice it can be a bit of a ghost town, with many businesses shutting down for long *vacances*. Holiday time in France is *très genereux* too, allowing for plenty of relaxation and time to unwind from the day-to-day grind of the office.

These gals set aside time on the regular to balance their work and personal lives, and to make sure they're fully present in both areas of their lives. "Parisian women will always take at least an hour per day for themselves and not run from meeting to meeting. We really try to balance. Work is not a priority for most of them," Leonor Greyl president Caroline Greyl explains.

But living a balanced life sure does top their list of priorities, and it definitely shows. "The Parisian lady pays attention to her lifestyle. She will take time to remove makeup, to clean her face, to use the right hair and face products, to go on a good diet, to spend time with friends, and to share good moments," Orlane General Manager Raffaella says.

LESSON LEARNED: WORK IS GREAT AND ALL AND IT'S AWESOME TO BE AN INDEPENDENT LADY BRINGING HOME A BIG PAYCHECK, BUT YOUR JOB SHOULDN'T BE THE END ALL AND BE ALL OF YOUR LIFE.

Having a life outside of the office makes you the cool, interesting person that everyone wants to be around, and gives you fascinating stories to share with good friends.

While we're on the subject of work, remember: Taking vacation time that you *earned* is a given, and it's just silly to let it go to waste. So take note from our Parisian pals and take a well-deserved break to de-stress from the workplace!

BEAUTY SLEEP 101: HOW TO CREATE A MORE RELAXING SLEEP ENVIRONMENT

Skimping on your beauty sleep? *Ooh la la!* A good night's rest is the hallmark of a well-balanced lifestyle, and *les Parisiennes* sure do know a thing or two about relaxation. They also know a good night's rest is a free way to get *très belle* skin. So no excuses! Can't seem to clear your mind at night? Lull yourself into a restful slumber and clock in more shut-eye with the help of these goodies.

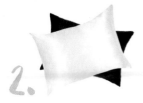

1.
SleepPhones® Wireless
Headphones in Quiet Lavender

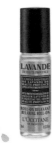

2.
Shhh Silk Pillowcase

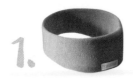

4.
Voyage et Cie
Boudoir Candle

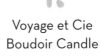

3.
iluminage™
Skin Rejuvenating
Eye Mask

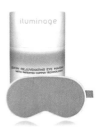

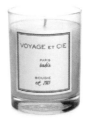

5.
L'Occitane
Lavender
Relaxing
Roll-On

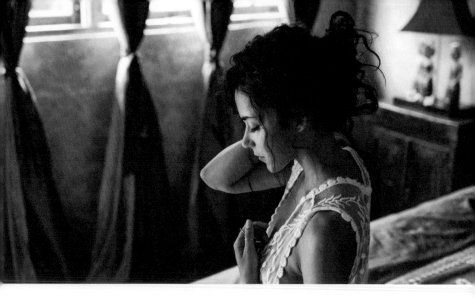

Dormez-Vous?

Feel like you're always burning the midnight oil? Been there, done that, *mes amies*. And if you've ever skimped on a night (or two or three…) of sleep, you know the end results aren't pretty when you wake up. The dark circles, the sagging skin, the hair that simply won't be tamed into submission—what a nightmare, right?

Sadly, sleep can sometimes seem like an indulgence for multitasking American women, and up until recently, the French were known for their envious sleep cycles. *Mais* stress seems to be catching up to even our European friends. "Like their American counterparts, French women now have sleeping problems due to stress," says Marie-Laure Fournier, a Parisian publicist based in New York City.

But the sleep-loving *beautés* of Paris put a high priority on rejuvenation and recovery, so they're able to bounce back from sleep issues pretty speedily. "The big difference is that we go more on vacations and weekend trips and therefore are able to recharge more often," Fournier continues.

If you're looking to get a bit more shut-eye and a bit less quality time with the wee hours of the night, it might be time to take a page out of Parisian ladies' books and put in for some vacation time—stat.

Taking some time out of your 9-to-5 lifestyle—even if you simply go on a long weekend trip—can be just what you need to jump-start your relaxing sleep cycle.

If that doesn't do it, maybe your quest for *parfait* skin will. Parisians are pretty religious about their anti-aging and skincare regimens in general, so clocking in a quality chunk of sleep (and washing off all that makeup beforehand) pretty much goes hand in hand with having gorgeous skin goals. Skipping out on sleep or their pre-sleep beauty regimen simply isn't an option for Parisian beauties who want to maintain their glowing complexions.

While you're adding sleep goals to your list, make sure you're also checking off all your sleep basics—you know, create a relaxing sleep environment and unplug from devices before bedtime to encourage better sleep. Indulging in a relaxing bath before bed can also be a nice way to lull you into a restful slumber.

UNDER-EYE MASK FOR DARK CIRCLES

This refreshing under-eye mask is perfect for making those raccoon-like shadows go far, far away.

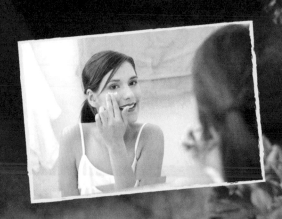

What Makes It Parisian?

French women aren't the greatest fans of heavy concealer... hence they're constantly on the lookout for natural remedies that do away with the need for heavy cover-up.

What Does It Do?

All these ingredients are potent sources of Vitamin K, which heals damaged capillaries and minimizes the pooling of blood under the eyes – the main causes of dark circles. Over time, it also thickens the skin around our eyes. And since thinner skin equals more visible dark circles, it's a powerful 1-2-3 punch.

Ingredients
1 bunch basil
1 bunch parsley leaves
3 lettuce leaves
3 cabbage florets
2 cups water

1. Boil the water and add the remaining ingredients.

2. Simmer for 20 minutes, then strain the liquid and pour it into a glass jar.

3. Apply this liquid (once it's absolutely cool) with a cotton ball under the eyes and leave on for 10 minutes.

4. Finally, rinse and gently pat dry; repeat daily.

5. This mixture must be refrigerated; discard if it smells rancid.

Rejuvenating Lavender Toner

This lightly scented toner feels super fresh and leaves skin radiant.

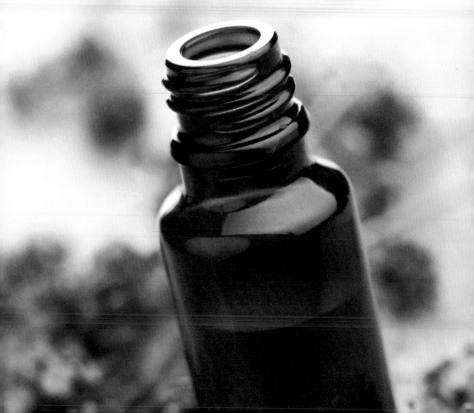

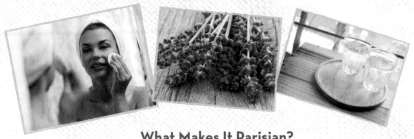

What Makes It Parisian?

Aside from it being *lavande*? Parisian women swear by toners
as a part of their beloved skincare routines.

What Does It Do?

Lavender is known for its circulation boosting properties.
This steps up blood flow, which in turn ensures adequate
oxygen and nutrition for skin cells.

Ingredients
Handful of fresh lavender
100 ml distilled or spring water

1. Bring the water to a boil.

2. Pour in the lavender, making sure it's completely
submerged.

3. Cover the bowl and leave the brew to steep for
a few hours.

4. Drain the mixture.

5. Pour the water into a clean glass bottle and store
in the refrigerator; use as a toner every morning after
washing your face.

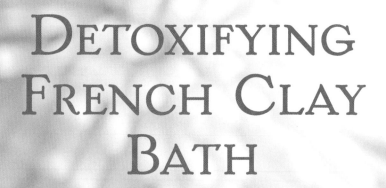

DETOXIFYING FRENCH CLAY BATH

This therapeutic bath will leave you feeling lighter and smoother.

What Makes It Parisian?

French green clay is a prized cornerstone of Parisian beauty.

What Does It Do?

French green clay literally binds to toxins, drawing out impurities and heavy metals from the body. At the same time, it's chock-full of minerals, which makes it extremely nourishing for the skin.

Ingredients

1 cup French green clay
1 cup Epsom salt
1 cup apple cider vinegar
10 drops lavender, jasmine, or rose essential oil
Small glass bowl

1. Pour the French green clay into the glass bowl and mix with warm water until you get a soft paste (this will stop the clay from clumping up in the bath).

2. Run the bath water, making it as hot as you like.

3. Pour this paste into the bath water.

4. Add the remaining ingredients and agitate to dissolve everything together.

5. Soak for 20 minutes; rinse off with a hot shower.

BATH AND BODY PRODUCTS
FIT FOR A PARISIAN

Bathing beauties? Parisians definitely wrote the book on how to bathe in style. With a bath-loving culture that spans centuries, these gals know a thing or *deux* about how to primp in the tub. Emulate their relaxing routine with these bath and body treats.

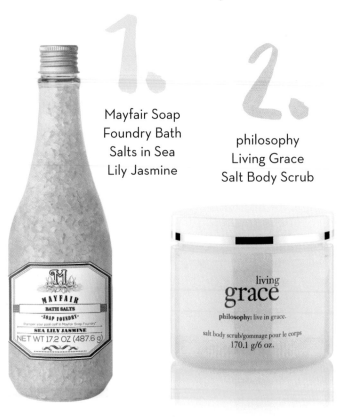

1.

Mayfair Soap Foundry Bath Salts in Sea Lily Jasmine

2.

philosophy Living Grace Salt Body Scrub

3.

LALICIOUS
Sugar Lavender
Hydrating Body
Butter

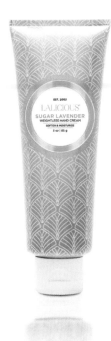

4.

Moroccanoil
Dry Body
Oil

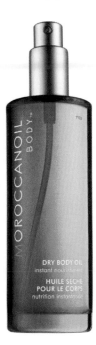

5.

John Masters
Organics Lemon
& Ginger Hand
Cream

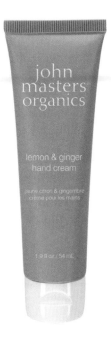

ROSE WATER HAIR RINSE

This utterly beautiful floral water will leave a very delicate scent in your locks long after you rinse it out.

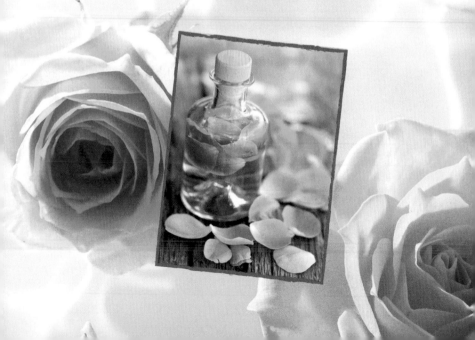

What Makes It Parisian?

French women have been great believers in beauty waters ever since Marie Antoinette stocked Versailles with gallons of *eau de rose* (rose water) and *eau de bleuet* (cornflower water).

What Does It Do?

Rose water normalizes hair's pH balance, repairs damaged cuticles, busts dandruff, and treats scalp inflammation.

Ingredients

6 cups organically grown rose petals
Distilled water
An enamel pot

1. Wash the rose petals completely and remove all the leaves and stamen.

2. Fill the bottom of an enamel pot with rose petals.

3. Pour distilled water over them until they are just covered.

4. Heat the water until it starts steaming but don't let it come to a boil.

5. Simmer until the petals lose their color. At this point, the water will have taken on the color of the petals and you will see oil on the surface. This will take approximately 60 minutes.

6. Strain the water and squeeze out the liquid from the petals.

7. Add half a cup of this liquid to a mug of water; use this mixture as a final rinse after shampooing and conditioning your hair.

Bathing *Beautés*

When you think of luxurious bath routines and the trendsetters behind them, French women should definitely pop up in your mind. These *chic* chicks have been setting bathing trends for centuries, whether or not they even realized it—just think back to the days when wealthy French women would sit back and let others bathe them! If history is any indication, it's safe to say that the French sure do appreciate the art of bathing.

"Historically, bath is not only a relaxation moment but also a sign of luxury. The first women who were able to have a bathtub in their house were all from the upper class. And remember, centuries ago you were bathed," Fournier says.

HISTORICALLY, BATH IS NOT ONLY A RELAXATION MOMENT BUT ALSO A SIGN OF LUXURY.

While Parisians approach the art of bathing a bit differently these days—ya know, women bathe themselves in the privacy of their own tubs—the relaxing nature of the process hasn't changed for the French culture, and women cherish a range of luxurious bath products that serve multiple purposes.

"We still very much love to bathe in France and we have many products for different purposes because bath can also be therapeutic (when you have skin problems or bone problems) or also help you lose weight (this is why you bathe with seaweed, for instance, at a certain temperature)," Fournier explains.

Some of their product faves? Foaming products and salts are two popular items, but these bathing beauties don't discriminate when it comes to their product routine. Any product that smells good, feels luxurious, and comes in multiple varieties—healing, relaxing, toning, etc.—rate highly among Parisian ladies.

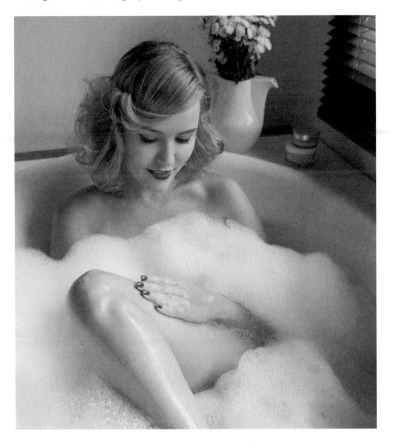

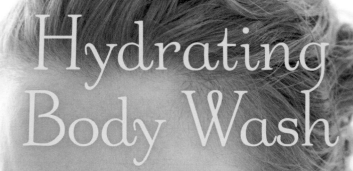

Hydrating Body Wash

This mild, beautifully scented, and slightly tingly body wash is the perfect good morning treat for your body and mind.

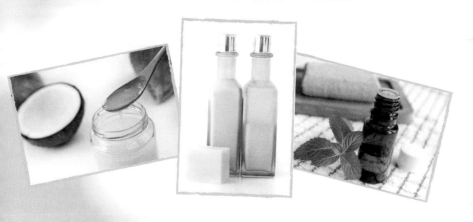

What Makes It Parisian?
Harsh cleansers are an absolute no-no for French women.

What Does It Do?
The hydrating and nourishing properties of rose water and coconut oil, combined with the natural soap base, will leave you sparkling clean without drying the skin. Peppermint oil makes for a perfect pick-me-up with its cooling and energizing effect.

Ingredients
2 cups liquid Castile soap
(or any unscented organic body wash)
1 cup rose water
4 tablespoons coconut oil
20-30 drops peppermint essential oil

1. Pour all the ingredients into a bottle and shake until everything is mixed well.

2. Shake before every application and use as a body soap.

MUSTARD BATH

*Soaking in a hot mustard bath
is a traditional remedy for
tight, achy muscles.*

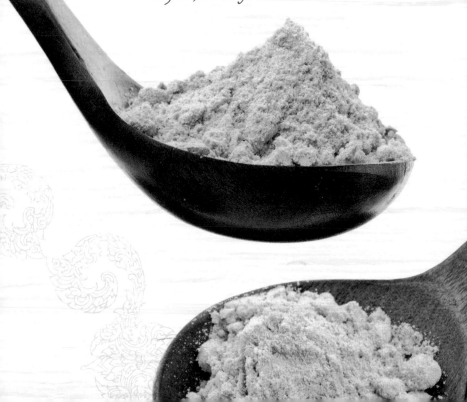

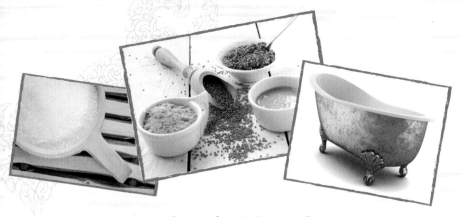

What Makes It Parisian?
French mustard has a cult status in both culinary and beauty genres.

What Does It Do?
Mustard has healing compounds that draw out toxins, improve circulation, relax tight muscles, and speed up the healing of damaged tissues.

Ingredients
2 cups Epsom salt
¼ cup baking soda
¼ cup dry mustard powder
6-8 drops eucalyptus essential oil

1. Mix together all the ingredients and add to hot running water.

2. Soak for 20 minutes, then rinse well.

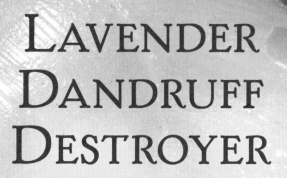

LAVENDER DANDRUFF DESTROYER

The relaxing scent of lavender will stay with you long after you've washed away the oil!

What Makes It Parisian?

Parisian women are known for their signature no-fuss hairstyles. They achieve this through natural, organic potions rather than the chemical-based ones that leave hair dull and brittle.

What Does It Do?

Lavender oil rejuvenates the follicles, thereby encouraging hair growth. It also kills lice and dandruff; regular use can improve your hair texture.

Ingredients

15 drops lavender essential oil
2 tablespoons olive or almond oil

1. Mix together all the oils.

2. Microwave the mixture for about 10 seconds or until it feels warm.

3. Massage the oil mixture into your scalp and through slightly damp, towel dried hair.

4. Put on a shower cap (to retain the heat) and leave for at least an hour; shampoo and condition as usual.

Lavender Body Scrub

A slightly gritty scrub that smells delicious and is great for soothing and relaxing the mind with the powers of aromatherapy.

What Makes It Parisian?

It speaks to the dual French love for simplicity and aromatherapy.

What Does It Do?

Lavender contains powerful antioxidants, which counter the effects of environmental pollution on the skin. It also keeps acne-causing bacteria in check, while increasing cellular rejuvenation and boosting the circulatory system, thereby increasing the flow of oxygen and nutrients to skin cells. Oatmeal and baking soda both make for great manual scrubs that are simultaneously soothing and hydrating.

Ingredients

1 cup dried lavender flowers
2 cups whole oatmeal
$\frac{1}{2}$ cup baking soda
Food processor or blender

1. Place all the ingredients in the food processor or blender.

2. Grind until you have a smooth, fine powder with the consistency of whole grain flour.

3. Store in a dry, clean container.

4. To use, slightly wet the powder and use it to scrub your body, paying special attention to rough areas like elbows and knees.

SCALP SCRUB

Try this gritty scalp scrub once a month for a healthy scalp and glossy strands.

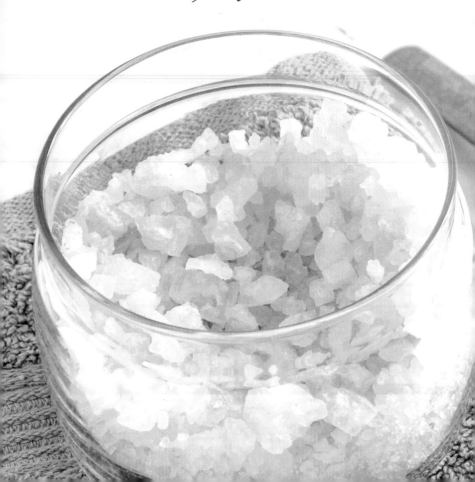

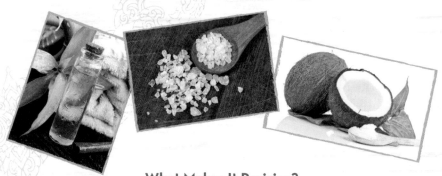

What Makes It Parisian?
Because Parisian women hate residue-laden strands.

What Does It Do?
Exfoliating your locks helps banish nasty product buildup that can clog and weigh down hair follicles. It also clears dead cells, attacks scalp acne, boosts circulation, and eliminates flakes.

Ingredients
3 tablespoons coarse sea salt or raw sugar
3 tablespoons coconut oil
4-5 drops tea tree essential oil

1. Lightly mix the salt or sugar with the coconut oil; don't blend so much that the granules dissolve completely.

2. Add the tea tree essential oil and mix again.

3. Wet your scalp and then massage it in gentle, circular movements with this mixture for a couple of minutes; then shampoo and condition your hair normally.

Grooming *Habitudes*

You know that stereotype about hairy French women who walk around with unkempt body fuzz? Banish it from your brain because they actually take grooming quite seriously; they just approach it a bit differently than we do!

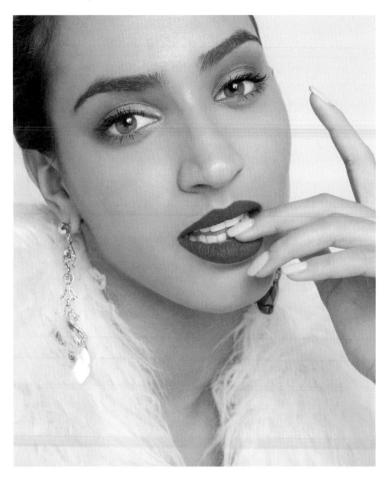

For instance, did you know that razors are a rare find in Parisian women's beauty cabinets? Yep, they mostly prefer waxing to shaving and it's not surprising either, considering the fact that it's so easy to get the service performed at local spas. "It's cheaper to get waxed in France than it is in America because it's more common," Anne-Cecile Curot, the French founder of Le Visage Spa in Boston, says.

Regular trips to their favorite day spas for waxing services are a *nécessaire* part of Parisians' monthly spa routine, but there's one area they avoid waxing: the eyebrows. When it comes to eyebrow grooming, tweezers are their tool of choice, and Parisians love to get their brows shaped. "We don't wax eyebrows in France, we tweeze. We shape them so it takes a little longer," Curot reveals.

Beautifully shaped brows are, of course, one of the trademarks of the Parisian makeup look, and they add instant polish. With look-at-me brows, you really don't need much makeup at all, so it's not shocking that Parisians take the time to carefully shape theirs.

LESSON LEARNED: SOMETIMES, THE SLOWEST GROOMING TECHNIQUES CAN PRODUCE THE MOST STUNNING RESULTS.

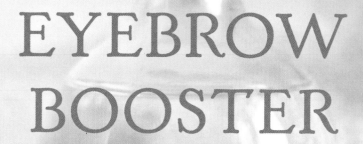

EYEBROW BOOSTER

*This silky blend sinks
right in and is perfect for
use before bedtime.*

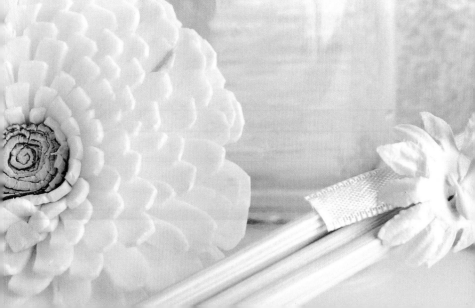

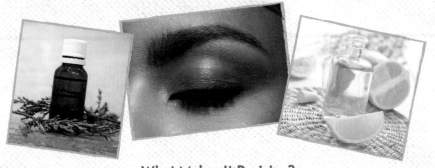

What Makes It Parisian?

Parisian women love a well-defined brow but don't like using too much makeup or artificial fillers.

What Does It Do?

The oils in this blend nourish fragile eyebrow hairs and their underlying follicles to boost growth and maintain the color.

Ingredients

1 teaspoon lavender oil
1 teaspoon rosemary oil
1 teaspoon thyme oil
1 teaspoon pine oil
1 teaspoon sandalwood oil
1 teaspoon lemon essential oil
1 teaspoon olive oil

1. Mix together all the oils; store in a glass bottle.

2. Massage this mixture into your eyebrows daily, before going to bed.

INDULGENCE IN MODERATION:

The *Délicieux* Parisian Diet

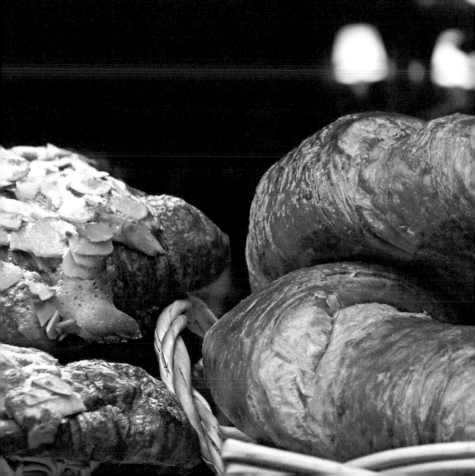

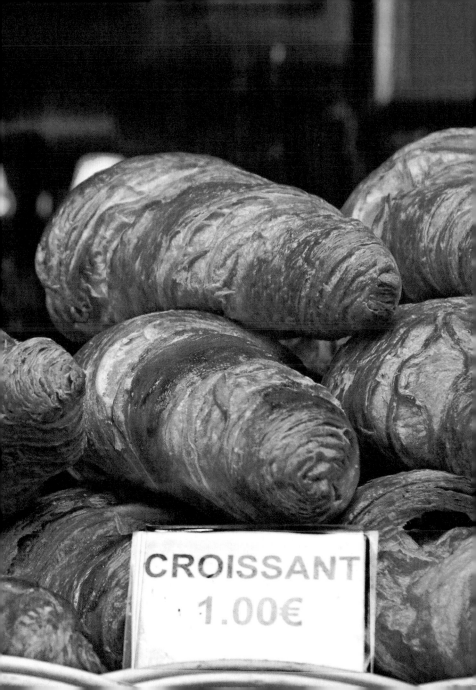

CROISSANT
1.00€

T ake a stroll down one or two Paris streets and you'll soon notice a bit of a culinary trend: *boulangerie, pâtisserie, fromagerie,* repeat. Bread, pastries, and cheese, oh my!

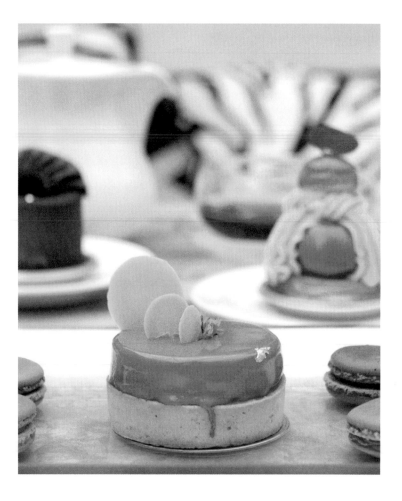

THE FRENCH DEFINITELY AREN'T IN THE HABIT OF SELF-DENIAL WHEN IT COMES TO ONE OF LIFE'S GREATEST PLEASURES, AND YET THEIR WAISTLINES DON'T SEEM TO SUFFER FOR IT.

Let's be honest, ladies, if we didn't love them for it, we'd probably hate them!

A lot of us tend to avoid cheese, bread, and pastries like they're the plague, but Parisian women indulge in these tasty goodies and much more without second thought, and don't apologize for it. So how do they enjoy all of the finer foods in life yet maintain trim waistlines? And what can you glean from their eating habits? Well, you've come to the right place!

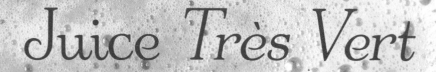

Juice Très Vert

The French have been locavores
since long before it was trendy in
the United States, always prioritizing
fresh, in-season, and locally sourced
produce from local open-air markets.
This healthy green juice recipe
is best made with local or
organic produce, like a true
Parisian would do!

What Makes It Parisian?

Don't be afraid to indulge in your favorite treats; just balance out your health regime with a mini-detox, like the French do. Swap in this juice for your usual breakfast or mid-day snack to soak up the nutrients and give your system some cleansing.

What Does It Do?

Leafy greens (especially dark ones) are a rich source of minerals, especially iron, calcium, potassium, magnesium, and vitamins B, C, E, and K — and even small amounts of omega-3 fats. These vital micronutrients will boost your metabolism and have you glowing from the inside out.

Ingredients

4 oz fresh spinach or kale (stalks removed)
1 apple, diced
1 cucumber, diced
4 celery stalks, diced
Fresh grated ginger root to taste

1. Put ingredients into a juicer or a blender, alternating greens with fruits and vegetables.

2. Pour into a glass over ice and enjoy!

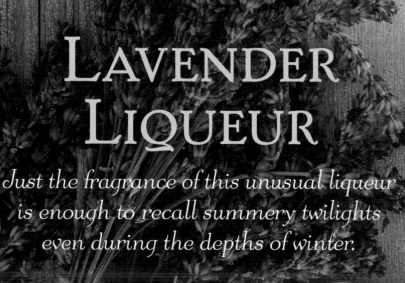

LAVENDER LIQUEUR

Just the fragrance of this unusual liqueur is enough to recall summery twilights even during the depths of winter.

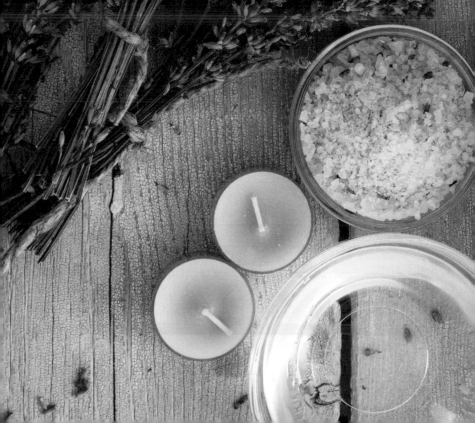

What Makes It Parisian?
It's lavender in a bottle! Enough said.

What Does It Do?
Taken internally, lavender tones the digestive tract, eases bloating, and flattens the belly. Its aroma is also perfect for soothing anxiety, calming the nerves, and focusing attention.

Ingredients
3 cups fresh, food grade lavender flowers
(or 6 tablespoons dried lavender)
750 ml bottle of 80 proof unflavored vodka
²/₃ cup sugar
Strainer or cheesecloth
Large glass jar with lid

1. Wash the flowers to remove all leaves, stems, and dirt; sort and throw away any that look damaged.

2. Leave them to dry in the sun for 1 hour.

3. Pour the flowers into the glass jar.

4. Add the remaining ingredients, stir, and cover the jar.

5. Shake mixture daily and let it stand for 2 weeks.

6. Strain away all the ingredients and pour the liquid into a sterile bottle; cap and store in a cool, dry place.

Clay and Honey Face Cleanser

This slightly gummy face wash is perfect for detoxifying your skin and getting rid of surface imperfections, like blackheads. However, it's not going to get off all that makeup, so you need another method (pure sweet almond oil works perfectly!) to do that.

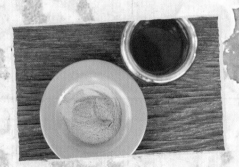

What Makes It Parisian?

Parisian women prefer gentle, organic cleansers to the harsh, chemical-laden products found on the market.

What Does It Do?

The super-absorbency of French green clay makes it effective at drawing out dirt, grime, grease, and all other toxins from the skin. The rice flour gives it the added benefits of a gentle scrub, while tea tree oil makes for a great antiseptic and antibacterial. Finally, raw honey not only hydrates and nourishes the skin, it also helps in the rinsing – if it's raw honey, you'll be surprised by how easily it emulsifies and slips off with just a bit of water, *sans* any stickiness or residue.

Ingredients

2 tablespoons French green clay
½ cup raw honey
½ tablespoon rice flour
5 drops tea tree oil
Small glass bowl
Small glass jar

1. Whisk together the honey and French green clay in the glass jar until you have a smooth paste.

2. Add the rice flour and tea tree oil; whisk again until everything is well-blended.

3. Scoop out the paste and store it in the glass jar.

4. To use, scoop out a small bit of the paste and apply to dry skin.

5. Rub it across the skin, using gentle circular motions for a minute; then rinse away with warm water.

Manger in Moderation

While French ladies love to eat, the Parisian diet is all about balance and healthy indulgences.

Marie-Laure Fournier, a Parisian publicist based in New York City, says French women approach eating in moderation so they can enjoy all of their favorites without sacrifice: "You can have a little bit of everything as long as it is in small portions. But when I go to Paris, usually you have appetizer, entrée, and cheese or dessert. They even created a new way to drink your coffee at the end of the meal to get a little bit of sugar and chocolate. But again, the portions are very small."

Getting to eat a taste of all your beloved treats, just in small portions? Sounds like an OK compromise to us! And it makes sense too, since the French are known for their leisurely meals with several courses. When you're indulging in course after course, the portions have to be *petite* so you can save room for the next *délicieux* surprise.

Lesson learned: No food should be "off limits." You can, and should, enjoy all the foods you want, just in moderation! They always seem to taste better when they're saved for a special treat anyway, don't you think?

YOU SHOULD ENJOY ALL THE FOODS YOU WANT, JUST IN MODERATION!

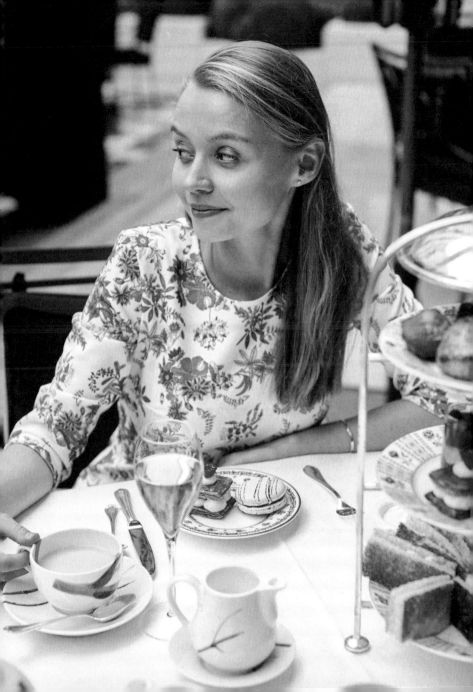

DEEP-CLEANSING CABBAGE FACE MASK

This leafy, deep cleansing face mask has the consistency of Russian salad!

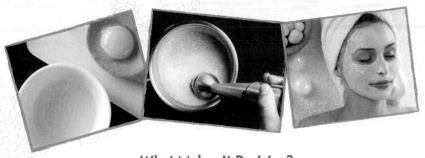

What Makes It Parisian?

Parisians are fairly obsessive about facial masks made from cabbage. In fact, so intrinsic is the Parisian love for cabbage that they have even made it a term of endearment ("*mon petit chou*" or "my little cabbage").

What Does It Do?

This leafy veggie is chock-full of sulphur and potassium, along with vitamins A, C, and E, which makes it wonderful at deep cleansing, evening out, and nourishing the skin.

Ingredients
Quarter head of cabbage
1 egg white

1. Grind the cabbage in a food processor or grater and put aside.

2. Beat the egg white.

3. Mix the cabbage and egg white together, blend well.

4. Apply this paste on your skin and leave for 20 minutes, then wash off with warm water.

Smoothing and Brightening Grape Face Mask

An indulgent treat that's perfect for smoothening and brightening the skin!

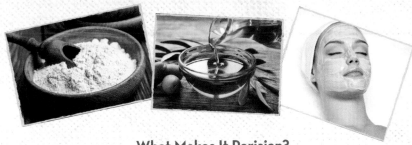

What Makes It Parisian?
The French love for grapes is legendary.

What Does It Do?
These juicy fruits contain loads of AHAs, antioxidants, vitamins, oligo-elements, and essential oils to improve circulation and step up hydration. You'll love the fruity aroma of this mask, and the results will leave your skin hydrated for days.

Ingredients
8-10 grapes (red or black are more potent than green)
1 teaspoon olive oil
2 tablespoons gram flour

1. Mash the grapes and transfer to a bowl.

2. Add the olive oil and gram flour to the grapes and mix everything well, until you get a thick paste-like texture.

3. Apply this paste to freshly cleansed skin then wash off with warm water after 15 minutes.

Natural Cherry & Pomegranate Brightening Peel

This natural peel may feel a bit tingly but it's perfect for brightening and firming the skin.

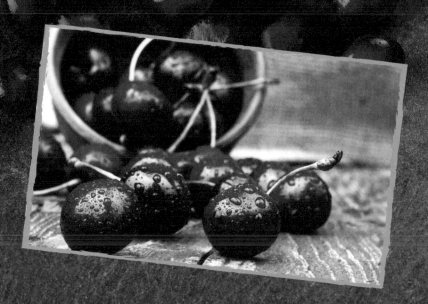

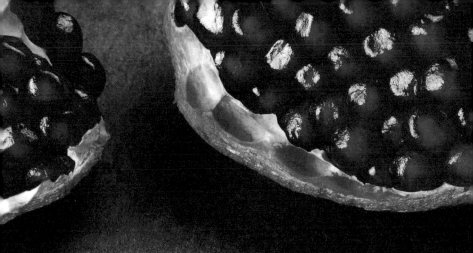

What Makes It Parisian?
It's an old Gallic recipe, dating back to the early 1800s

What Does it Do?
The natural enzymes help brighten and firm the skin, without the harsh side effects of chemical peels.

Ingredients
10-15 cherries, pitted
3 tablespoons pomegranate seeds

1. Mash together the cherries and pomegranate seeds (you can whisk them in the blender, on a low setting, for a smoother consistency).

2. Apply the paste on freshly washed skin, leave for 10 minutes and then rinse off with warm water.

5 FOOD RULES FRENCH WOMEN LIVE BY

Parisian women don't put many restrictions on themselves as far as their beloved eating habits go, but they do live by a few key dietary rules. Ready to eat like a *Parisienne*? Study their top five food rules.

1. Wine is always a good idea!

2. Never, ever rush through a meal.

3. There is no such thing as an "off limits" food.

4. Food always tastes better with family and friends.

5. Eat everything you want, in moderation.

Eating Slowly *Ensemble*

Sitting down to a tasty meal with multiple courses pretty much forces you to eat slowly and savor the food you're eating, instead of shoveling it down and rushing to your next task. "When we eat, we eat, we don't vacuum food," Anne-Cecile Curot, the French founder of Le Visage Spa in Boston, explains. "We enjoy cooking, we enjoy eating, we like to sit down."

When you're always running around to work or social activities and don't make time to focus on your food, you start to eat mindlessly. And a lot of busy gals find it challenging to even find time for a proper sit-down meal, never mind one with multiple courses. But Parisians make it a priority to enjoy every meal, even when at work. The French have long been known for their leisurely lunch breaks and taking the time to eat slowly allows them to actually feel full, enjoy their food, and digest.

Larger meals and richer foods that leave you full and satisfied for longer periods of time mean you don't need to frequently snack on junk food, either, and the French frown upon it, in fact. "Snacking is the biggest no-no in France," Fournier says.

Eating with *les amis* or *la famille* also helps, of course, and meals are a big communal time in France. Long, relaxed meals are par for the course for Parisians and they enjoy the good company almost as much as they enjoy the yummy food. Almost!

"Food is part of the DNA in French culture. We grow up around family meals—that's where and when you meet around the table and share your day, your life, your issues, and your meal with your loved ones," says Elisabeth Holder, co-president of Ladurée US.

FOOD IS PART OF THE DNA IN FRENCH CULTURE.

From setting the table to enjoying a meal together, the whole process of eating is a ritual that French women have perfected, and instead of rushing through the process, they prefer to savor every single moment. "I think the French value the time it takes to prepare a meal. It's sharing that moment with friends and loved ones that creates a meal," Holder explains.

GRAPE AND CLAY HAIR VOLUMIZER

This slightly gritty hair mask will give you healthy, shiny, bouncy hair.

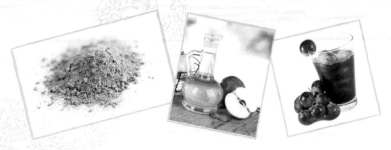

What Makes It Parisian?

This recipe combines natural clay and grapes – two of the most French ingredients in the universe.

What Does It Do?

Clay helps remove the excess oils that make hair look limp and dull. Grapes feed the scalp with antioxidants, while helping to gently polish away dead skin cells.

Ingredients

2-3 cups grape juice
1 tablespoon white clay
1 cup green tea
2 tablespoons apple cider vinegar

1. Combine all ingredients in a glass bottle and shake well.

2. Shampoo your hair as usual.

3. Pour this mixture liberally over wet hair, then massage lightly into scalp and along your hair length.

4. Allow to remain on your hair for a minute, then rinse off with cool water.

5. Towel dry your hair and style as usual.

EAT YOUR WAY LIKE A FRENCH WOMAN ACROSS THE USA

Can't make it to Paris anytime soon but dying to get a taste of their tempting treats? Good news! You can *manger* your way through the United States like a Parisian with these authentic French delicacies in a town near you.

1. LADURÉE

The Famous French bakery has two locations in New York and one in Miami so you don't have to fly all the way to Paris to get a taste of their *délicieux* macarons.

2. LA MAISON DU CHOCOLAT

Share Parisians' *amour* for chocolate? These popular Paris chocolate boutiques have locations in New York City and New Jersey, or you can have their goodies shipped to you anywhere in the United States and beyond!

3. TARTINE BAKERY & CAFÉ

Make sure you stop into this San Francisco hot spot on your next trip to California! From French breakfast faves to tasty desserts, sandwiches, and wine, Tartine has treats for every mood.

4. AUGUST

A trip to New Orleans is like a tiny taste (literally) of France, especially when you dine at August, one of the city's hottest French restaurants located in the Central Business District.

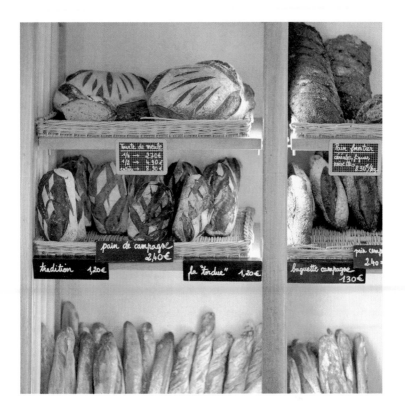

Favorite French Foods

What tops the list of their food essentials, you ask? It'll come as no surprise, but French women love bread! Baguettes, bread, and croissants are three of their go-to options for breakfast (although they try not to indulge in the latter too often!), in fact, and they love to spread jam, marmalade, or butter on them to add a little extra flavor. Parisian women get their morning jolt of caffeine from *café au lait* and black coffee, but in general, they don't take their coffee cups to go, and would rather sit down to really enjoy them.

For lunch, meat and veggies are usually the dishes *du jour*, so you'll find these healthy diet staples stocked in *la cuisine* of French women. You'll also find rice and pasta (served in small portions), fresh cheese, fruit, and asparagus. They love to steam the latter and pair it with a béchamel sauce or homemade vinaigrette for a tasty appetizer. Tomato salad or shredded carrots with a homemade vinaigrette are two other appetizer faves. Mmm, mmm, we're getting hungry already!

The rumors are true, and dinner is served in courses, so come prepared with an appetite! If you indulged in a big lunch, dinner usually consists of lighter fare to maintain the idea of moderation. "The rule in general for women is that if you had a heavy lunch you dine with a soup. We love soup in France," Fournier reveals.

They also love their cheese, of course, but don't eat it in bulk, and typically pair it with pears or lettuce. Fresh is the name of the game for Parisians, who are lucky to live in proximity to oodles of food markets, and they prefer fresh to processed foods, opting for home-cooked meals or dinner at a local bistro over takeout. Traditional French dishes like *foie gras* are of course faves, but are often saved for special occasions like holidays.

Naturally, wine is the preferred drink of French women, and it has some pretty strong health benefits, too, but they rarely drink just for the sake of drinking. "We love our wine, but usually we don't drink wine without food," Curot says.

Le vin isn't the only indulgence Parisian ladies appreciate; they also have a strong love for *chocolat* and *macarons*. "The macaron is something everyone indulges in not just as a dessert but as part of your day. It's a small beautiful treat," Holder says.

When they want a piece of chocolate or a *macaron*, Parisian ladies don't deny themselves the small treat, and we could definitely benefit from their laid-back approach to indulgence.

Manger and Moving

If you imagine French women magically subsisting on bread, éclairs, and wine and never gaining an ounce, you're probably not alone. Their carefree approach to eating is pretty badass, after all. But they're not magical unicorns who can eat all day long with no repercussions.

In reality, French women eat what they love, but they do so in moderation, and they move a lot to make up for the rich ingredients in their favorite foods. Parisian women rack up a lot of steps per day walking around the city — from commuting to work on *le métro* to making a stop at local food markets — and they don't put a high priority on actual gym time, so they make sure to move frequently throughout the day. "We're not big on working out. Not that we think it's stupid, but we're not obsessed with working out," Curot says.

Parisians are definitely not gym rats, but that doesn't mean they never work up a sweat! They enjoy yoga, Pilates, boxing, and Zumba to work off all those tasty treats they enjoy so much; they just aren't slaves to their routine.

So they don't deny themselves indulgences; they make the time to eat with family and friends; they truly savor their food; *and* they're not obsessed with working out? Sign us up for the Parisian diet, stat!

Bottom line: Forget the idea that you have to deny yourself—or exhaust yourself—to be healthy. Balance is the name of the game, and really, isn't that the way food and activity should both be enjoyed—with pleasure and in moderation?

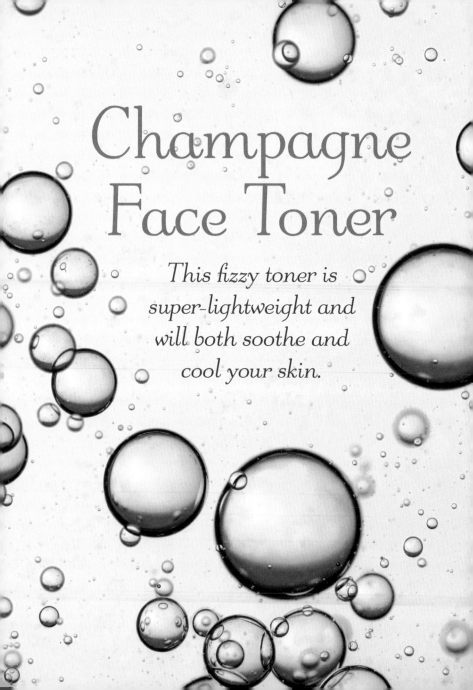

Champagne
Face Toner

This fizzy toner is
super-lightweight and
will both soothe and
cool your skin.

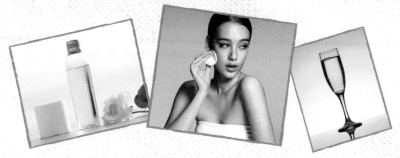

What Makes It Parisian?

Um . . . it's *champagne*! Traditionally, French royalty have bathed in bubbly, and this toner is a cult skincare treatment among French women.

What Does It Do?

Champagne (or sparkling wine) is loaded with antioxidants that halt premature aging and keep wrinkles at bay. It's also high in tartaric acid content, which is a known anti-bacterial and skin lightener that helps clear up acne, detoxifies the complexion, and busts hyperpigmentation. And that's not all: the bubbling action of champagne helps step up micro-circulation *and* constrict pores for that healthy, radiant glow.

Ingredients
Chilled champagne (or sparkling wine)

1. Soak a cotton pad in chilled champagne (or sparkling wine).

2. Wipe thoroughly across a cleansed face, neck, and *décolleté*.

3. Don't rinse off; follow with your regular moisturizer.

WINE BEAUTY PRODUCTS ALMOST TASTY ENOUGH TO EAT

Can't get enough of *le vin*? There's a beautiful way to extend the fun of this tasty treat. Beauty products colored in the rich hue or infused with resveratrol are an ideal option for the à *la mode femme* who loves a glass of red every now and then.

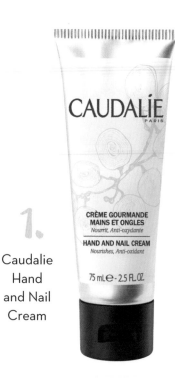

1.

Caudalie
Hand
and Nail
Cream

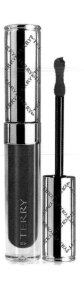

2.

By Terry Terrybly
Velvet Rouge in
My Red

3.

ZOYA®
Nail Lacquer
in Dakota

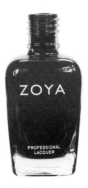

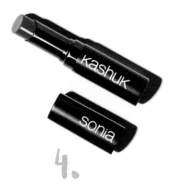

4.

Sonia Kashuk®
Moisture Luxe
Tinted Lip Balm in
Hint of Berry

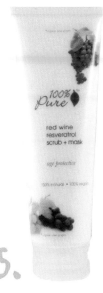

6.

Hourglass
Femme
Rouge®
Velvet Crème
Lipstick in
Icon

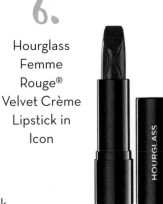

5.

100% Pure® Red Wine
Resveratrol Scrub + Mask

ORANGE BLOSSOM WATER TONER

Moist, green, and cool, this orange flower water will transport you to sunny orange groves even on the muggiest of days.

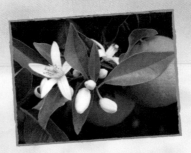

What Makes It Parisian?

Bitter orange trees have long been cultivated in France to produce orange blossom water.

What Does It Do?

Orange flower water makes an excellent toner for delicate, sensitive, and oily skin as it is a good astringent, is antibacterial, and can soothe overheated or sensitive skin. Its scent is also uplifting, refreshing, and helps dispel tension and stress.

Ingredients

4 cups orange flower petals, preferably
organic and from bitter orange trees
Distilled water
Strainer or cheesecloth
Mortar and pestle
Large glass jar with lid
Small sterilized glass jars with lids

1. Wash the flowers to remove all leaves and dirt; sort and throw away any that look damaged.

2. Leave them to dry in the sun for an hour.

3. Using the pestle and mortar (or any other blunt instrument), grind the petals to release their natural oils; let this paste-like maceration sit for a few hours.

4. Pour the macerated petals into the large, lidded glass jar.

5. Add approximately one cup of distilled water per 25 petals; when in doubt, use less water as you can always add more later.

6. Close up the jar and let it sit in the sun for about a month. After this, check the scent; if it's too weak, leave the jar out for another week.

7. Strain away the flower petals, pour the liquid into sterilized, lidded glass jars, and store in the refrigerator.

RED
WINE
BATH

*This dreamy, floaty bath will
nourish the mind and soul
as much as the body.*

What Makes It Parisian?
Vinotherapy, which is based on the health
and beauty benefits of grape extracts,
was born in France.

What Does It Do?

Red wine is packed with resveratrol and other polyphenols, powerful antioxidants that counter premature aging, inflammation, and sun damage. Epsom salts regulate the activity of over 325 enzymes, reduce inflammation, help muscle and nerve function, prevent the hardening of arteries, improve the absorption of nutrients, and flush out toxins. Grape seed oil is full of antioxidants and essential fatty acids that prevent and reverse environmental damage, minimize skin aging and help control acne. Finally, honey is a great detoxifier and natural humectant (an element that attracts moisture and locks it into skin), which restores hydration and elasticity to the deepest layers of your skin.

Ingredients

½ bottle red wine
(day-old wine is absolutely fine!)
½ cup grape seed oil
1 cup honey
1 cup Epsom salt

1. Pour the red wine into a warm bath.

2. Add the Epsom salt.

3. Pour in the honey and grape seed oil just before you get in the tub.

4. Soak for 20 minutes.

INDEX

CREDITS

CHAPTER 1

SIDEBAR: STOCK YOUR BEAUTY BAG LIKE A PARISIAN PRO

Photo Courtesy of Yes To, Inc.
Photo Courtesy of bareMinerals
Photo Courtesy of L'Oréal Paris
Photo Courtesy of tarte Cosmetics
Photo Courtesy of Urban Decay
Photo Courtesy of Votre Vu
Photo Courtesy of Laura Geller

SIDEBAR: 5 STEPS TO THE PERFECT PARISIAN RED LIP

Photo Courtesy of eos™
Photo Courtesy of Burt's Bees®

SIDEBAR: 6 SIMPLE STEPS TO A TRÈS CHIC FRENCH LOOK

Photo Courtesy of Joanna Vargas
Photo Courtesy of BECCA
Photo Courtesy of Physicians Formula
Photo Courtesy of Kevyn Aucoin
Photo Courtesy of FLOWER
Photo Courtesy of Paul and Joe Beauté

SIDEBAR: ROCK FLAWLESS PARISIAN SKIN WITH THESE 6 SKINCARE SAVIORS

Photo Courtesy of Yon-Ka Paris®
Photo Courtesy of Vichy Laboratoires
Photo Courtesy of First Aid Beauty®
Photo Courtesy of IXXI
Photo Courtesy of Darphin
Photo Courtesy of SkinCeuticals

CHAPTER 2

SIDEBAR: SPA CHEZ VOUS: HOW TO CREATE AN AT-HOME FRENCH SPA EXPERIENCE

Photo Courtesy of Paddywax®
Photo Courtesy of Lavanila
Photo Courtesy of Talika
Photo Courtesy of Clarisonic®
Photo Courtesy of Erborian
Photo Courtesy of Orlane
Photo Courtesy of Dr. Dot
Photo Courtesy of Marie D'Argan Paris
Photo Courtesy of OPI
Photo Courtesy of Oribe
Photo Courtesy of Dessange Paris

SIDEBAR: TRÈS CHIC TRESSES: PRODUCTS TO HELP YOU RULE THE PARISIAN HAIR GAME

Photo Courtesy of Kérastase
Photo Courtesy of Christophe Robin
Photo Courtesy of Leonor Greyl
Photo Courtesy of StriVectin®
Photo Courtesy of Alterna Haircare

CHAPTER 3

SIDEBAR: NEUTRAL IN *NOIR*

Photo Courtesy of ModCloth.com
Photo Courtesy of Anne Fontaine
Photo Courtesy of Old Navy
Photo Courtesy of Wren + Glory
Photo Courtesy of Loeffler Randall

SIDEBAR: LADY IN *ROUGE*

Photo Courtesy of Banana Republic
Photo Courtesy of Nicole Miller
Photo Courtesy of Ghurka
Photo Courtesy of Jean-Michel Cazabat

SIDEBAR: TRENCH CHIC

Photo Courtesy of Zady.com
Photo Courtesy of Abercrombie & Fitch
Photo Courtesy of Aquatalia
Photo Courtesy of Target
Photo Courtesy of DSTLD

SIDEBAR: 5 MUST-HAVE ACCESSORIES FOR TIMELESS PARISIAN STYLE

Photo Courtesy of Lacoste
Photo Courtesy of Mangrove
Photo Courtesy of Dr. Scholl's Shoes
Photo Courtesy of JustFab
Photo Courtesy of Jemma Sands

CHAPTER 4

SIDEBAR: BEAUTY SLEEP 101: HOW TO CREATE A MORE RELAXING SLEEP ENVIRONMENT

Photo Courtesy of AcousticSheep LLC
Photo Courtesy of Shhh Silk
Photo Courtesy of iluminage™
Photo Courtesy of Voyage et Cie
Photo Courtesy of L'Occitane

SIDEBAR: BATH AND BODY PRODUCTS FIT FOR A PARISIAN

Photo Courtesy of Mayfair Soap Foundry
Photo Courtesy of philosophy
Photo Courtesy of LALICIOUS
Photo Courtesy of Moroccanoil
Photo Courtesy of John Masters Organics

CHAPTER 5

SIDEBAR: WINE BEAUTY PRODUCTS ALMOST TASTY ENOUGH TO EAT

Photo Courtesy of Caudalie
Photo Courtesy of By Terry
Photo Courtesy of ZOYA®
Photo Courtesy of Sonia Kashuk®
Photo Courtesy of 100% Pure®
Photo Courtesy of Hourglass

ABOUT THE AUTHOR

Chrissy Callahan is a beauty, fashion, and lifestyle writer. Her work has been published in both print magazines and online outlets, and she's covered everything from backstage beauty at New York Fashion Week to celebrity interviews. A proud Francophile, she loves traveling (especially to Paris!), reading, and all things beauty and style-related.

ABOUT THE RECIPE WRITER

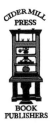

Anubha Charan is the blogger and beauty expert behind the hugely popular website TheBeautyGypsy.com. She has also worked as the Managing Editor for *Vogue*, the Beauty Director for *Marie Claire*, and a Beauty Editor at *Cosmopolitan*.

ABOUT CIDER MILL PRESS BOOK PUBLISHERS

Good ideas ripen with time. From seed to harvest, Cider Mill Press brings fine reading, information, and entertainment together between the covers of its creatively crafted books. Our Cider Mill bears fruit twice a year, publishing a new crop of titles each spring and fall.

CIDER MILL PRESS

BOOK PUBLISHERS

Visit us on the Web at
www.cidermillpress.com
or write to us at
PO Box 454
Kennebunkport, Maine 04046

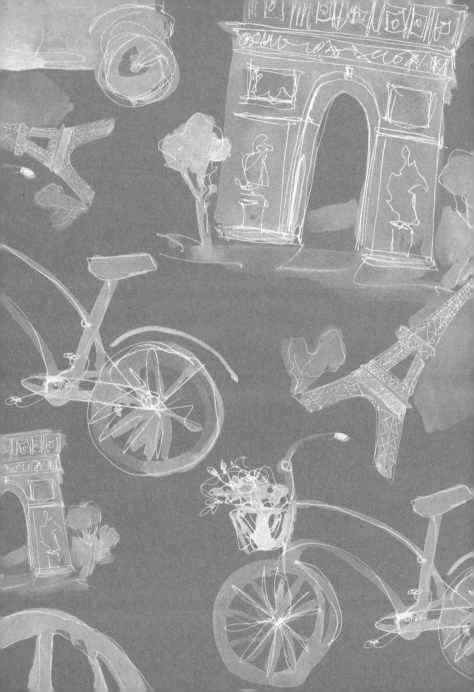